No Pity Party for Me!

The Girl Who Refused to Fail

Paula Leone Heulings
with Kathryn Ross

Pageant Wagon Publishing
Vineland, NJ

ISBN: 978-1-7360080-1-0
BIO026000   BIOGRAPHY / Personal Memoirs

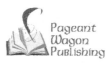
Pageant
Wagon
Publishing

Pageant Wagon Publishing
Collaborative Author: Kathryn Ross
Cover, Interior Design, and Formatting by Kathryn Ross

Dedication

This book is dedicated to my two sons,
David and Gregory,
and my grandchildren,
Sophia, Landry, and Emmitt.

May you always believe in yourself
and do all things fearlessly
knowing our good God loves you
and has great mountains for you to climb
with joy and celebration.

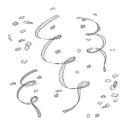

Acknowledgements

Thank you to my family and friends who have remained steadfast to encourage me through the years to write and publish my story. You know who you are and if I tried to list you all, it would fill another book. I might have left my story in pieces halfway up this mountain but for your continued support to complete the task.

Thank you to my husband for making the financial arrangements for this project. Your generosity, love, and support of what you knew was important to me, in such a tangible and necessary way, made this finished book a reality.

Thank you to my Beta Readers, Danielle and Kalee, for your generous time and unbiased feedback devoted to reviewing the original manuscript of this book prior to publication. Your thoughts and considered opinions were greatly appreciated in this publishing adventure.

Thank you to every doctor, nurse, therapist, and health care provider who ever poked, prodded, and pushed me beyond my limits to achieve my goal of healing and restored living. Apart from you, this book could never have been written, and this story might not have had a happy ending with PARTY!

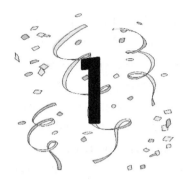

THUD!

"Quit fooling around," Alan murmured as he rolled over with a fluff to his pillow. "You getting David?"

Sprawled on the floor on the side of the bed and barely awake, the stabbing headache that had hounded me for the past two days exploded between my ears.

"Mommy! Mommy!" Our two-year-old, David, called out to me from his crib.

I tried. I really tried to move my legs. To will my muscles to flex and push me to stand. To walk.

To no avail.

Tears welled in my eyes out of frustration. Fear clutched my throat and choked me in sudden panic. My breath shortened in little gasps of dread, confusion, and staccato shrieks building to a blood curdling scream. The knife-sharp head pain intensified.

Alan sat erect, shocked wide awake. "What! Paula? What? Are you crying?" He stumbled out of bed and around to the other side then looked at me laying there, helpless in a heap.

Something was very wrong.

"I can't get up! My legs won't work! Come to me! Do something!"

1

THREE DAYS EARLIER I'd celebrated my older sister's engagement. Marianne and her fiancé Dean decked out the yard at his parents' house on the water in Collings Lake, New Jersey for a big party.

The Sunday afternoon sun shone brightly over the festivities as adults played horseshoes while the kids ran about enjoying the grassy grounds. Old friends gathered for the event and sat together under shade trees. Dean's carefully compiled playlist of favorite tunes provided the background soundtrack featuring the chart-topping hit makers of 1986: Michael Jackson, Bon Jovi, and Whitney Houston. Lively chatter filled the air as everyone caught up on each other's lives.

Guests enjoyed a buffet of home-made salads, Mom's meatballs, and each family member's favorite potluck recipe. Harry, Dean's dad, grilled hamburgers and hot dogs over charcoal flames. The scent wafted through the yard awakening everyone's appetite.

Crowned with a huge sheet cake in honor of the happy couple, the dessert table featured my famous ambrosia and my oldest sister Susan's signature cream puffs. The sweets and salads were magnets for all manner of flies, gnats, and a bee or two, even though we made a valiant effort to keep the food covered throughout the humid summer afternoon.

The day wore on as Marianne and Dean opened their gifts—including a total of three toasters—to a chorus of approval. They thanked their guests for coming. The food, fun, and games eventually drew to a close.

Most of the friends and relatives left as the late afternoon shadows fell, but a few stragglers wandered to the end of the dock overlooking the lake. Alan and I watched our toddler son David play in the sand and weeds nearby. We laughed at his cute attempts to skip stones at the edge of the water with PopPop Vince—my father.

"Ouch!" Marianne slapped her shin. "Nasty mosquitos."

Dean put his arm around her and pouted playfully. "Awww. 'Cause you're so sweet, Mair."

My husband, Alan, put his arm around me and laughed. "Say, Dean—how about we take the boat out before it gets dark?"

"Good idea! Hey, who wants to go for a sail?" Dean jumped into the boat and started to prep for some late-day fun on the water. "This is the perfect way to close out the party."

"I'm in!" I said, and confidently climbed aboard with Mair and Alan.

I believed myself to be a professional sailor. After all, I went to summer camp throughout my teen years and learned to sail on the challenging waves of the Chesapeake Bay. Marriage and motherhood did not quell my adventurous spirit. At nineteen and the baby in the family, I took on the responsibilities of adulthood early when I married before my middle sister. I held down a day job in a hair salon and worked towards my beautician's certificate at night, kept home for my husband, and faced the demands of toddlerhood undaunted. My energy and enthusiasm for life remained youthful and fearless. Like an intrepid kid I was usually up for anything that smacked of fun and enterprise. Knowing David was safe with mom and dad for an hour or so, a late day jaunt on the water after our all-day party was right up my alley.

"I've got the rope over here, Dean! Ready to cast off when you are!"

The small Sunfish with its blue and white striped sail slid away from shore, cheered on by some of our remaining friends who waited on the dock. We took turns heading out since the boat could only hold four at a time. Being the expert sailor, I was determined to play first mate to Dean as captain for each trip. Alan and I waved at David and PopPop, who were joined by Mom at the edge of the water.

I breathed in the fresh air and lifted my face to the gentle breeze as we skimmed over the lake. For the first few moments we remained silent, just enjoying the comfort of the rocking boat and lapping of the waves against the sides. Eventually, our conversation turned to wedding planning ideas with lots of laughter and cheerful hope for the future.

Dusk fell too soon, and we made our way home on the last sail around, tied up at the dock, and stepped back on shore. I ran off to get David from my mother who had put him to work on clean-up detail gathering balloons and streamers. He took immediate possession of his treasures with glee.

"Still plenty of clean-up to do," Mom said. "Many hands make light work." She pointed to the trash bags and tables that needed clearing.

We all pitched in. The guys folded up tables and chairs while the kids gathered trash. I grabbed empty salad bowls and brought them into the kitchen where Mom had suds up to her elbows rinsing everything in sight.

"Just put the bowls on the table, Paula. I'll get them in a minute," she said. Then her brows furrowed as she looked close at me. "Ooo, what's that huge welt on your shoulder?"

"Welt?" I twisted my neck to the left to see where she pointed. Yep—there was a welt, alright. "Probably just a mosquito bite. There were tons of them out there. I'm surprised we weren't eaten alive."

We slept soundly that night after a long, fun-filled day.

The next morning it was back to the daily routine. Alan and I readied ourselves for work and I dressed David to take him to my parents' house for the day. "I want to take my balloons, Mommy," he said, holding three helium balloons tight to his fist.

"Fine. Fine." I had no desire to argue with a toddler. I felt a sudden surge of weakness and tried to shake it off. *Must have overdone it yesterday!*

But by the time we arrived at Mom's house, my head stung with a piercing pain. I'd never known a headache like that before and had to sit down on the couch.

"You okay, hun?" Mom said.

"Yeah. Just a headache. I'll be fine in a minute." I'm good." I planned to sit down for only a minute or two. Then exhaustion overtook me, and I had to lay down. I never made it to work that day.

Instead, I slept for hours. When mom woke me she found that I had a slight fever. She made chicken soup and I drank a little broth before heading home. *What a weird day!*

After persevering through the splishy-splashy bathtub ritual with David, I put him to bed and crawled under my own covers, still nursing my headache.

By morning, when the headache hadn't subsided and I still felt awful, I headed for Dr. Haag, our family physician. Someone had canceled earlier so they fit me right in.

"Looks like a sinus infection." Doc Haag wrapped up my case in no time, prescribed antibiotics, and sent me home.

I didn't go to work at the salon that day, but there was plenty of work to be done around my house: beds to make, random organizing to do, and mommy-time toddler games with David. The normal home routine moved along smoothly enough, despite my nagging headache and the mosquito welt on my left shoulder that remained mildly annoying.

A mosquito bite. THE mosquito bite.

The mosquito bite that changed my life.

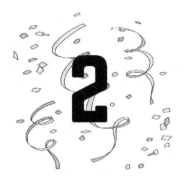

"I can't get up! My legs won't work! Do something!"

Alan ran to my side of the bed where he saw me sprawled in a panic. Still in a morning stupor, he helped me to the bed. "What's the matter, babe?"

My panic ratcheted to shrieks and gasping sobs. "My legs won't work! I can't feel my legs!"

I heard his soothing words to me, but he was scared. His hands trembled and fumbled with the phone and his voice cracked as he explained our situation to the 911 operator. I saw the concern in his eyes as he hung up the receiver. "The ambulance will be here soon. It's going to be okay."

Somewhere in the mass of confusion in my mind, I thought of David. *I need to get David!* Things went a bit foggy, and a flood of helplessness washed over me.

The few minutes it took for the EMTs to arrive felt like hours. I was aware of great commotion—image wisps of faces and colors and movement swirled around me as though I were watching a movie, unable to interact.

Then, darkness.

Beeeep! Beeeep! Beeeep!

A small army of nurses rushed to my side and ordered me to be still. "Settle down! Settle down! Hush, hun!" Arms forced against my upper body in a vain attempt to still me. They pushed me down into a bed with metal rails like a prison.

"Where am I? What's going on? Let me go!" Flail! Flail!

I'd awoken from a semi-coma, in shock at my alien surroundings. Wires and cords connected me to strange machines with flashing lights and shrieking alarms. I panicked at the sight of it all—threatened—and reacted like a mad woman. I ripped cables, tape and whatever I could grab in a frenzied attempt to escape.

A very solemn nurse strapped me to the bed. "Settle down, miss. You don't want to be a problem patient."

Exhausted from my fit, I watched her secure me and wipe my forehead. *Problem patient?* "What happened?"

"Your mother and husband are outside. I can send them in if you promise to be still. Doctor will be in soon." She spoke in a firm, measured tone. No nonsense.

"Alan? Mom?" I tried to sit up, but a stern look from the nurse settled me in place. She exited from my view with a promise to return.

Mom and Alan stepped into the room. At the sight of them sobs bubbled to the surface. "Paula! Shhh. Shhh, honey." Mom stroked my hair standing over me on one side of the bed.

"Hey babe?" Alan smiled. I saw relief flush across his face, mixed with the sense of something else I couldn't quite determine.

"What happened? Where's David? I need to get David?" *I want my baby. Where is my baby?*

8

"David is fine, hun," said Alan. "He's with mom and dad. He's just fine." I understood that to mean that David was with Alan's parents. They often helped with babysitting since we both worked. *David is fine. Good. But what about me?*

"Will someone please tell me what I am doing here?" My memory focused. "I was just at home. Got out of bed, and . . ."

Mom squeezed my hand. "Sweetheart, you've been in a semi-coma for a couple of days."

"Days?" I struggled to remember more. Then suddenly, "My LEGS!" Mom held tight to my hand. Alan clasped the other. "I . . . I can't feel my legs."

In a matter of minutes, I learned the whole story. Two days of my life were missing from my memory due to the coma, but not, apparently, from a company of doctors and nurses poking me, prodding me, and syphoning blood from me with all manner of x-rays. They hooked me up to a host of bells and whistles to stabilize my body functions and ran a battery of tests to determine what had caused my condition—including a test for Guillain Barre Syndrome, a paralysis resulting from allergic reactions to a shot.

Once awake, all I could do was I lay in bed and wait for a diagnosis while nurses came and went, in a daily routine to check my vitals and draw blood for more tests. And more.

Visits from family—and especially my precious little David—were a high point of those long, few days. I'd never been so bored. So inactive.

Eventually, my room turned into Grand Central Station with visitors dropping by with well wishes and prayer promises. People's faces, in and out all day, blurred together so I couldn't keep track of them. I only know they visited because Mom told me.

My room swiftly filled with balloons, flower baskets and stuffed animals to cheer me. The party atmosphere of the room was meant to distract me from the sterile hospital monitors, cables, and that bothersome IV drip. I really hated being tied down to an IV drip.

As a matter of fact, I really hated everything about being in that hospital room. The incarceration wore me down emotionally, and I struggled to maintain any semblance of courtesy. I became that problem patient the nurse had prophesied me to be—and warned me against.

"Someone needs to shave my legs!" I demanded one morning while another faceless and nameless nurse checked my stats. "All these people coming to see me. It's embarrassing."

After a bit, another nurse entered with a little shaving kit and lathered up my legs. I couldn't feel a thing. I watched, helpless, and wiped a tear from my eye. *I wish I could feel how soft and cool the shaving gel is!*

I didn't want to look weak, so I forced a stern expression on my face. Then, I saw it. Little red lines. Cuts and scrapes from the razor. The nurse sliced me during the shave in more than one place. I couldn't feel it, so I didn't cry out in pain. I surveyed the damage after she left. *Maybe I should have just left them hairy. What a mess! That's gonna leave a scar—I just know it!*

But, by far, the worst thing I had to acquaint myself with that first traumatic week was the pee bag. My paralysis from the waist down meant that my bladder didn't work either. Just the thought of a catheter threaded up my you-know-what made me shiver. *Catheters and pee bags are for old people. Right?*

"Can someone empty that pee bag?" I commanded an unassuming orderly who'd dropped in to remove my food tray. "It's disgusting."

"I'll see what I can do," came a mousy reply. I'm sure I scared her, Problem Patient that I was. She looked pretty young—like me. Young and walking, though, with plans go to the movies later. Or shopping. Or maybe even a road trip with her friends to Great Adventure—my favorite amusement park. It was only a couple hours' drive away. *Drive! I bet she drives, too! You have to be able to feel the pedals to press them just right to drive. I . . . I can't drive anymore!*

Little by little, grave thoughts materialized in my understanding as the gravity of my situation fell upon me like an elephant on my chest. The elephant in the room that everyone else already understood. Whatever my condition, it was dire and serious.

Even so, still no diagnosis. Or prognosis.

The nurse entered to check my pee bag hanging off the side of the bed. "Paula, the bag's not full. It doesn't need emptying every time there's a little drop in it."

"It's gross. I hate it."

She checked my vitals again and ignored my snarky reply. "Your parents are here. They'll be in to see you in a bit." She smiled and left the room, all cheerful and perky.

I hate cheerful and perky.

The door remained ajar, and I could hear voices in the hall—Mom and Dad, and the doctor. Straining to hear their conversation in hushed tones, I could only pick up a few words here or there. Then, a startling phrase sent me into another panic.

As I tried to wrap my mind around what they were discussing, Mom and Dad's voices grew louder, and they entered the room—cheerful and perky. "Hi, sweetheart! How are you doing today?" Mom said.

I shot back, "What do you mean, my head is swollen and has a greenish cast?"

The color drained from Mom's face and all cheerfulness faded. She and Dad exchanged furtive glances. They were hiding something from me. *I'm paralyzed from the waist down. Is there something worse they haven't told me yet?*

"Oh, Paula," Dad said, "you weren't supposed to hear that."

"I'm paralyzed. Not deaf, Dad."

Mom looked grim, "Well, dear, the truth is, there's a bit more to your injury."

At that point, Marianne waltzed into the room with a singsong, perky lilt in her voice, "Hiya, baby sister! What's up?" But after one look at our grave expressions, her countenance fell. Something serious was afoot.

"Your sister wants a mirror." Mom said.

"A mirror? Are you sure?" Marianne drew closer to the bed.

"Do you have one in your purse?" Dad asked.

"Just my compact." Marianne lifted her fringed leather bag.

"Let me have it!" I stared her square in the eye with my demand.

Marianne looked for direction from Mom and Dad. All her perk melted away.

What is wrong with me that they know? That Alan knows? That the doctors and nurses know? That everyone who has visited me probably knows? Except me? I held out my hand to Marianne for the mirror. "Hand it over."

She pulled out a little Revlon compact—the one we bought a couple of weeks ago when we went shopping for bridal makeup ideas.

"Now, dear," Mom said, "The doctor assures us it won't last. Really."

I grabbed the compact, opened the lid, and raised it in front of my face. Even through the powdery residue I could finally see what everyone else saw. Not believing it to be true, I wiped the mirror clear and looked again. The elephant in the room that weighted my chest. I should have kept the powdery veil in place.

My head was swollen. Swollen big. I didn't even recognize myself. And even worse—a greenish tint had replaced the youthful, fresh-faced complexion I'd always been so proud of. "I look like an alien!"

Fresh tears flowed among the four of us. *Wake me up! Wake me up now, God! Will this nightmare ever end?*

Once the emotions in the room settled, they explained that the swelling and green color was a result of water on the brain from the infection.

Infection?

There was an infection. An infected mosquito bite. I still felt the pain from the welt on my shoulder. But what did that have to do with not being able to move my legs, go to the bathroom, or looking like an green alien?

They meant well to hold back full disclosure of my condition. But I had to know it all. Dad explained the details and next steps. "The doctor is coming in later today to do one more test. A spinal tap. To examine the fluid at the base of your spine. We hope to have some answers after that."

"Fluid on my spine?" I thrust myself back against my pillow. "As if water on the brain isn't enough!"

"It's all related, Paula," said Mom. "You're my strong girl. You can do this! We'll have answers soon. Everything will be fine."

"Will I get to go home soon?"

An awkward pause followed. Mom avoided my question and changed the subject. "How about Dad and I head down to the cafeteria to get a treat? What do you want us to bring you? I'm afraid we finished the last of Marianne and Dean's cake from the party. Sorry."

I didn't care about eating party cake. I had no appetite and didn't want a treat. I didn't feel very strong, either. What I did want was to be well and be home with my Alan and David and get back to my normal, healthy life.

Marianne sat on the edge of the bed after Mom and Dad left. We chatted about nothing for a few minutes before Dr. Haag walked in carrying a metal bin. "How's our Paula today?" He tried to be chipper.

I hate it when doctors try to be chipper.

As he proceeded to explain about the spinal tap test, Mair backed away from the bed into a corner near the door while a nurse prepared me for the simple procedure. I looked at my sister and motioned for her to stay when I saw her eyes widen in fear. "Oh, my goodness!" she gasped.

"What?"

Mair grimaced and mouthed words in a low tone and animated fashion. "It's-a-good-thing-you-can't-feel-anything-because-that-needle-is-this-long!"

She positioned her hands about 18 inches apart before the nurse stepped between our line of sight and ushered her out of the room.

I closed my eyes. *I'm a healthy, young woman who is never sick. I have a little boy to take care of. This must be a dream. A terrible dream!*

"Now," said Dr. Haag, "this won't hurt a bit. Really."

God! End this nightmare!

I don't know if it was days or hours before Dr. Haag returned with Alan and my parents to discuss his findings. I'd spent the early portion of the week in a semi-coma and the latter portion of the week trying to process the horrifying change of fortune in my life.

The tests resulted in a diagnosis of Post-Infectious Encephalomyelitis. An infected mosquito bit me. The bacteria that caused the infection passed into my bloodstream and through my system. There was no medication they could give me because the bacteria no longer existed in my system. Only the effects of the attack lingered. It did its damage and left me paralyzed from the waist down. We listened to him in shocked silence.

"The fluid in your brain will drain. Your swelling will go down. You'll lose that alien pallor and be back to your pretty little self soon. However," he paused. My heart sank. A sick sensation surged through the part of my body, and I wanted to shut out whatever he might say next. "I'm afraid the paralysis is permanent. You will never walk again."

The paralysis is permanent! I will never walk again! How is this possible? God? Okay—this has to be a dream. A nightmare even. Just not real! Please! This can't be real!

But I wasn't sleeping or dreaming. I was wide awake, and it was real. I had just lived through the scariest moment of my life. There had to be better days ahead . . . right?

15

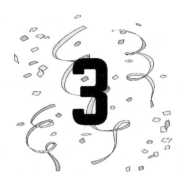

They're talking about me. I know they're talking about me. But I couldn't hear what they said.

The doctor took my husband aside just out of earshot. Mom and Dad stepped closer to hear the low-toned conversation. Marianne sat on the bed with tears in her eyes as she watched them.

"What? What is going on? What are you talking about?" I raised my voice to arrest their attention.

Mom stepped back to my bedside and patted my hand. "Don't worry, dear. We're gonna figure this thing out."

Figure what out? I strained to listen and caught random words: Living arrangements . . . ramps . . . wheelchair . . . handicapped accessible . . .

Handicapped? I'm HANDICAPPED!

"Hey! Talk to me. What are you discussing? I need to know."

The doctor looked at me and smiled. "Just a few instructions for when you go home, Paula."

"You're releasing me?"

His stone-faced expression didn't change. "Just a few more things to look into on that."

"What do you mean?"

Mom tried to calm me. "Now, dear, settle down. We're going to get it all figured out." Her eyes brimmed with tears as Marianne held back her waterworks, too. Their attempt at bravery in the face of my dire diagnosis did not encourage me.

Instead, something else welled up from deep within me. I had no need to fight back tears. Anger surged to the surface of my emotions, with a desire to fight back against the words I heard bantered about in my room: *Handicapped accessible. Bathroom fitted for handicap. Doorways adjusted for handicap. Handicap! Handicap! Handicap!*

I don't know how my chaotic mix of volatile passions settled, but eventually I lay quiet and alone in my room. I absentmindedly counted the bizarre faces I saw in the pocked ceiling tiles above me—like so many demons laughing at my predicament.

My imagination ran away with me like an old silent movie reel. Faded images of all my hopes and dreams flashed across the screen of my mind with swift, unnatural movements before they dissolved and faded to nothing. I tried to reach for them, to see them again, but they were gone.

Handicap. I had no time to be handicapped! I had a child to raise. A home to keep. A husband to love. And a new career to launch. There was no room on the calendar of my days for being handicapped; resigned to live the rest of my life in a wheelchair. *Nope. Just not happening!*

Except it was.

Over the next few days, I endured treatments to reduce the swelling and fully stabilize me, clueless as to what would happen next. Nurses, orderlies, and doctors came and went in routine fashion throughout the day.

Visitors stopped by to offer their support and assure me that they were praying for me. I learned to smile and say "thank you" even though their words rarely touched me with hope. I shut down.

Hospital staff congregated in my room and talked about me like I wasn't there. Doctors examined me then stood by the door to discuss amongst themselves what their next move might be. *What am I? Some kind of freak no one wants to deal with?*

Two weeks after arrival at the hospital, I stabilized sufficient for the next stage of the journey. "We've done all we can do for you now," they announced. "We're not sure how we can be of further help. You'll need to be transferred to a larger hospital."

"Larger hospital? You mean I'm not going home?" I turned to look blankly out the window. *Going from one prison to another. Is that really the best you can do for me, God?*

Alan and my parents worked together with the staff to get me properly placed in a choice hospital where, they assured me, I could recover enough to go home. Apparently my "numbers" weren't quite right yet for a safe release.

"It won't be for long, hun," Alan tried to encourage me. "You really are coming along well. And, besides, I need time to get things ready at the house."

"Oh, right," I sneered at him. "You mean all those special fittings for someone who is HANDICAPPED!?"

I immediately regretted my harsh words. He was only following the doctor's instructions for my wellbeing over the long term. The look in his eyes cut me and for the first time since I'd entered my horror movie, I thought of how someone else felt. "I'm sorry, Alan. I'm just . . . so sorry."

There were no words left to speak and nothing to do but wait to hear updates from the complex world of insurance companies, paperwork files, and organizing the physical transport of a patient from one hospital prison to another.

Over the next couple of days, we learned that my insurance did not cover the hospital selected for transfer because I had newly signed on. They categorized me with a pre-existing condition and refused to pay. *Yeah. Right. Like I knew this was going to happen.*

Mom made it her mission to storm the castle for justice. In hindsight, I can see where my fight club attitude came from. She got on the phone to the governor's office. Yes—the governor's office. If anyone could make the hospital accept me, it would be him. "No worries, Paula," she said with all the confidence of a fully armored warrior. "Remember, people are praying for you. We'll get these mountains moved."

But the doctors didn't put much hope in those prayers, or her petition to the governor's office. They looked elsewhere to line up other options.

But all things do work together for good, and God has a way of making the right things happen at the right time for all the right reasons. Even when we can't see the sense of it all and may not like the circumstances at first, He is faithful and in due season delivers the reward.

After a couple weeks of phone calls and paperwork, the insurance company capitulated, and the first-choice hospital accepted me. *Good on you, Mom! Thanks, God.*

In the meantime, though, the doctors completed all the necessary hoop jumping to get me into a different hospital—the Alfred I. duPont Children's Hospital in Delaware.

A children's hospital? Really? I'm a married woman with my own child. Well, okay, so I am just nineteen years old and technically still a teenager.

Apparently, that was a plus for me. Being six months shy of my 20th birthday, Alfred I. duPont accepted me.

The day before transfer I asked for a shower. After weeks of sponge baths in the hospital bed, I felt like I needed to be hosed down. My greasy hair needed a good scrubbing. Two nurses put me in a wheelchair and rolled me down the hall to the shower room. We walked in—wheeled in—and they turned on the water. They did not leave. Three of us there for one shower. In that instant, it hit me: *I AM an invalid. Oh, God! How can this be? I can't even give myself a shower?*

I wanted those two nurses to leave so I could get naked and wash. Alone. Like a civilized, healthy person. But no, they stayed. They had to stay. I was incapable of washing myself. It was humiliating.

I'd always been so independent. I married young, had a baby, husband, and a home to keep. Plus, on top of all that, I held down a job and attended classes, halfway through my training at beauty school to fulfill my career goals.

Right. Beauty school.

That was an oxymoron since I'd never felt so ugly and so utterly dependent, and incapable of doing the simplest self-hygiene chore.

I tried to wash what I could even though my left arm was a little weak. My hair. Armpits, Front torso—the nurse had to do my back. And legs. And feet.

"I can do that." I insisted. But no. I really couldn't do that. This was no ordinary bath time. I was naked, in a shower, in a sitting position with a catheter hanging out of my privates, hooked up to other wires, IVs, and monitors and four foreign hands manipulating body parts, soap, and washcloths on me. *Will this really be the rest of my life?*

After the shower, they rolled me back to my room and dressed me. Did you get that? The nurses dressed me. Like a little fashion doll. I couldn't even put on my own clothes.

Once I was properly positioned in bed again, they left me alone in my room. Staring at the pocked demon faces in the ceiling again. Solitary with my thoughts between sudden rushes of uncontrolled sobs. The silence from heaven was tangible.

Is this my life now? Am I going to need someone to do everything for me? If I could, I'd have pulled my knees up to my chest and hugged them in a fetal position, then cried myself to sleep. But all I could do was lie there. Flat on my back. And drift off to sleep on a tear-stained pillow.

Morning comes early in a hospital. At 6:00 a. m., the night shift made their last rounds before turning things over to the day shift. They woke me up, took my vitals, emptied the pee bag, and asked if I needed anything.

"Yes. I need something." I spoke, slow and soft. Then, like a cat taking its prey in a violent pounce, "I need my legs to work again!"

The doctors arrived to discharge me with great assurances of the excellent care I'd receive at my new hospital digs.

"Oh good, a place where they specialize in taking care of INVALIDS!" I snapped. I had no control over the harsh words and sentiments belched up from somewhere deep inside me. My only consolation was that I'd spoken under my breath, barely audible, if at all, to anyone else.

Though the nurses and orderlies who bustled about my bed and prepared to move me might not have heard it, I knew what I'd said and felt my heart. I winced in condemnation.

You are better than this, you know, Paula. It's not their fault. You know that.

The EMTs arrived, one of whom was a friend of our family, Mrs. Cook. "Well, you look much better than the last time I saw you."

"The last time?"

Her confident smile comforted me. "Our team brought you to the hospital from your home. But I guess you wouldn't remember that."

"No," I said, as they strapped me to a gurney. I glanced back into the room that had been my home for two weeks, then forward into the hallway as the EMTs wheeled me to the ambulance.

Alan sat by my side with Mrs. Cook for the ride while Mom and Dad followed in their car. It was a 40-minute drive out of New Jersey, over the twin bridge into Delaware, on the way to the new hospital. The new normal of my life.

Alan asked questions about the complex equipment in the ambulance and Mrs. Cook tried to keep the trip upbeat with random conversation about things I couldn't care less about.

My mind drifted.

Delaware.

I was familiar with the trip. I'd traveled NJ Route 40 West across the Delaware Memorial Bridge many times in my 19 years. Every summer for seven years, between the ages of 11 to 16, Mom and Dad drove me through Delaware into Maryland for my annual stay at a Christian Summer Camp in Sandy Cove. My last summer there, I spent more than two weeks in counselor training and tucked away some of the most cherished memories of my youth.

I loved the outdoors and had a voracious appetite for action and adventure. Exploring the wilds of nature was a particular passion.

That last summer at Sandy Cove, with Donna, Jennifer, Kristin, and Paula—yes, another Paula—we spent a week hiking the Appalachian Trail, carrying everything we needed to survive on our backs. The following week we canoed down the Susquehanna River. Camping out. Sleeping under the stars. Trading secrets by the fire into the dark nights. Waking to the sound of birds singing. Suiting up for new discoveries on a new day.

My legs were strong. I welcomed the challenges of every step I took, empowered by deep breaths of fresh air while I drank in the glories of God's creation.

One day we accidentally wandered into an old farmer's apple orchard. He scared us by shooting a rifle into the air. Talk about feeling close to God! Later, we explained ourselves and made friends. He sent us on our way with some delicious apples. Good times.

We made time daily for prayer and Bible study, but I felt closest to the Lord when I could sneak away to marvel in wonder at the mountains. How great and grand I saw God in the majesty of the wooded peaks, clean air, wide blue skies, and the peace that surrounded me there. I was so small. So small. Yet when I walked in intimacy with God in the guise of Creation, I learned to see and sense the tangible nature of His character—just like I'd read about Him in His Word.

Summers in Sandy Cove. And early September in Florida.

Ever since 8th grade, I'd gone to Florida with Alan and his family after Labor Day. We had been middle school sweethearts who married by high school graduation. My Florida happy place was Sea World where I indulged my obsession with dolphins—my go-to therapy animal.

Great memories.

But just memories. *This summer, clearly, will be different. And what about next summer? And the summer after that? And that?*

I wondered what Donna and Jennifer and Kristin and Paula were doing with their summer. Bet they were enjoying adventures with legs that actually worked. *Maybe they're at Sandy Cove with plans to hike the Appalachian Trail. I hope Donna doesn't miss me too much on the hike—if that's what she's doing this summer.*

Because we had different levels of fitness, I always hung back with Donna on our hikes. She struggled with the physical demands of the climb and threatened to quit even though she had set a personal goal to fulfill all the requirements to become a camp counselor.

Donna just needed a cheerleader, and I had enough energy to lend her the support necessary to get over the obstacles of the challenge. "You can do it, Donna!"

"No, Paula," she huffed, leaning against a tree. "You go on. I may just turn back. It's too hard. I'm not cut out for this."

"Nonsense," I said. "Just breathe. And step. Breathe. And step. You've got this!"

"But it hurts! And I'm soooo tired. I don't know what made me think I could do this counselor stuff. I'm not strong like you."

"You are, Donna! Believe it! You are Wonder Woman! You're great with the kids and they love you. And you have such a heart for others. You'll do anything for anybody. You're a good friend. That's what's really important to being a counselor."

"And being able to hike trails and row boats. It's the outdoor athletic stuff that I just can't manage."

"Well, that's where I come in. Two are better than one."

"Isn't that the memory verse from Ecclesiastes?"

"Yes. And if you get God in the middle of your struggle, it's a three-fold cord that won't be easily broken."

Donna caught her breath and laughed. "You're not going to leave me. Are you?"

"Nope," I said. "And neither will God."

Beeeeep Beeeep Beeeep . . . Whoop Whoooop Whoooop!

"What happened?" The ambulance came to an abrupt halt and shocked me out of my trip down Memory Lane. My eyes focused on a cramped space with harsh, blinking lights all around—far from the wide blue skies and rolling peaks of the Appalachian Mountains.

"No worries," said Mrs. Cook. "Just traffic. We're almost there. It's so congested here."

Alan agreed. "Yeah, we're pretty used to the boonies in South Jersey."

That 40-minute drive seemed like the longest in my life. Since I'd been in the hospital, everything took longer. Simple things dragged on. In slow motion.

What does it matter—stuck in traffic? I have all the time in the world, now. Nothing to do. Just wait.

But what was I waiting for?

When we arrived, Mom and Dad stood outside the ambulance entrance to greet. Automatic doors opened to welcome us as they escorted me across the threshold of my new home. Away from home.

"This looks very nice," Mom looked about at the cheery surroundings with approval.

Lying flat on a gurney I couldn't see much. While rolling down the hall I did notice that everything looked new and clean. There were a lot of paintings on the walls. Bright colors and childlike art decorated the hallways. Busy nurses and doctors hurried here and there.

We arrived at my room, and orderlies lifted me into a new bed in a private room with a private bath. *Hmmm. Too bad I can't really enjoy it since I can't pee or shower by myself.*

A large picture window overlooked an outdoor play area surrounded by beautifully tended, lush green grass. *Oh! Green grass in summer! Will I ever feel the tickle of cool green grass on my feet, again?*

After I settled in, some of the nurses dropped by to introduce themselves. Since this was a children's hospital the staff seemed friendlier than where I'd come from. They answered my questions about the hospital and told me a little history of the duPont Children's Hospital that diverted my attention from myself for a few minutes.

The duPonts were a fascinating crew—one of America's billionaire families dating back to the 19th century. They wanted to keep their money in the family and intermarried to secure their fortune.

Unfortunately, familial intermarriage often results in children born with mental illness, retardation, or severe handicaps. The duPont family built the hospital for their own children's maladies. Strange but true.

Everyone seemed genuinely kind. Most of my nurses were women except for one male nurse named Brian—kinda young and cute, with blond hair. Another woman named Paula (a name I could easily remember) had short, dark hair, old enough to be my mother. She proved to be a comfort to me with her calm, confident manner.

Mom, Dad, and Alan stayed a while to be sure I was okay before heading home. They had a 45 to 60-minute trip back to New Jersey.

As two nurses bustled around the room and settled me into bed, I noticed Mom rummaging around in her purse. She pulled out something stringy looking and stepped cautiously to my side. "I want you to keep these here with you." She opened her hand to reveal Rosary beads and a Scapula.

"What's this?"

"A Rosary to remind you that I have the whole eastern seaboard praying for you, and the Scapula blessing that protects you from death."

"Mom!"

She looked away for a moment as if to collect her emotions. I sighed as I noticed her eyes brim with dampness and an intensity I'd never seen before. I hurt. But my mother hurt, too. It was an awkward, yet tender moment shared between us. *How would I feel if I was standing over my David in a hospital bed with a stunted future?* "The whole eastern seaboard, Mom?"

She smiled and unfurled the Rosary and Scapula. "Well, a good bit of it." The clickity-clackity of the beads brushing one against the other reminded me of gentle windchimes—a transporting sound that I welcomed. She reached behind my head to drape them on a wall hook just above me.

"Thanks, Mom." I couldn't think of anything else to say.

Dad stepped forward. "Well, today was a big day. Let's go so she can rest."

It was late and a long drive home for them. We said our "goodnights," traded hugs and kisses, and they were gone so I could rest. *Rest? That's all I do.*

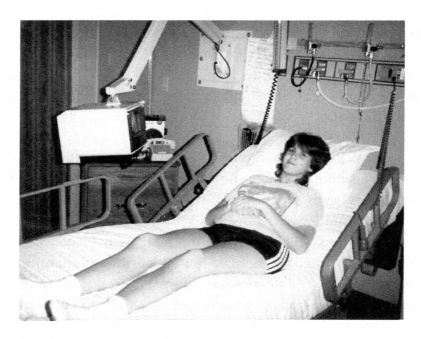

Look behind my pillow and you'll see one of the Rosaries that my mother hung from the medical equipment panel. Eventually, two Rosaries and a Scapula hung there as a constant reminder that the Lord was with me, and people were praying for me.

They promised to be back the next day. And the next. And the next. In fact, we swiftly fell into a routine of every-evening visits after their collective workhours.

A nurse dimmed the lights after they left, and I lay alone in a building with total strangers. Alone and depressed. Nothing on TV interested me to distract my thoughts.

Soon I drifted off to sleep and dreamed about hiking the Appalachian Trail. Canoeing the Susquehanna River. Standing—yes—STANDING on a hilltop overlook taking in the beauty of the Lord in the mountainous Mid-Atlantic landscape. *Will I ever be able to stand there again?*

And somewhere, deep down, I heard Donna's voice on that trail as if a prayer, "You're not going to leave me . . . are You?"

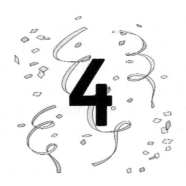

"Good morning, Paula, your breakfast is here!" A bubbly voice greeted me as I awoke after my first night at duPont. I had wondered what awaited me there. Breakfast was a good place to start.

As a merry little aide raised my bed so I could sit upright to eat, I took in the visual elements of my room. It was nicer than where I'd been before and featured a wooden dresser under the picture window that looked out on the hospital yard. An end table to the right of the bed gave it a homier feel.

To the left, behind my bed and just past all the hooks, wires, and flashing lights of hospital equipment, was the private bathroom. An oxymoron since I did not foresee myself ever able to use it privately. There would always be at least one person to assist me in toilet rituals going forward. Or so they told me.

Strategically placed opposite the bed, like seats in a theater facing the stage, sat a couple of industrial grade hospital chairs. One of them reclined into a makeshift bed for overnight guests. The only light in the room came from either the window or the glaring overhead fluorescent fixtures. *Well, I'll have to do something about that! This personal space needs to be . . . personalized.*

"There ya go!" The cheery aide conveniently adjusted the swivel meal table so I could reach my meal. She was about my age. "Is there anything else I can get for you?"

I held my tongue for the snark that might escape and shook my head. "No. Thank you."

"Okey-dokey! Enjoy!" She seemed to bounce from the room, happy and carefree, on two healthy legs.

I looked at the food tray setting before me and sighed. No silver breakfast service here. Just a nasty old fiberglass tray with a warming lid over industrial strength cafeteria dishware. I lifted the lid expecting the worst—if not mediocre fare. To my delight, the scrumptious scent of fresh, real eggs, warm toast, and hot coffee greeted me. The meal tasted as good as it looked and smelled. "Hmmm," I mused aloud with the first bite of a bright orange sunny-side-up egg, "that's yum. No accounting for presentation, though."

As I ate, I took in more details of the institutional ambience of my room. *Well, if I'm gonna be stuck here, I might as well try to make this place a bit more interesting to look at.*

The vase of flowers from Alan looked lonely on the dresser by the window, so I made a mental list of items to spruce things up a little. *I want framed pictures of Alan and David, and maybe a bowl of potpourri. It might help to mask the disinfectant odor in here. And this lighting has got to go. I bet Mom has a dresser scarf and can dig up a decorator lamp for the end table. Something to make it feel softer and more intimate at night.*

The staff gave me a few minutes to eat before both the happy little orderly and a young man entered my room. The former removed the dirty breakfast dishes and the latter introduced himself. "Hi, Paula! My name is Vinnie. I'm your physical therapist. Welcome to duPont!"

Why is everyone in this place so danged cheerful?

I tried to be agreeable in return. "My dad's name is Vincent."

"Well, then," he said, "you won't have a problem remembering my name, will you? You're going to be meeting a lot of people here, over the next few days. We plan to keep you pretty busy."

He did not lie. He was only one of my therapists. Later that day, I also met Karen, my occupational therapist. Both therapies were designed to strengthen and train me to become functional enough to go home and begin the rest of my life confined to a wheelchair. But we didn't do much that first day other than evaluate my condition in order to create a treatment plan.

Other than meeting my two therapists, the first full day of my stay at duPont included a doctor's exam, a tour of the hospital, and visits from the family after dinner. That was more activity in a twelve-hour span of time than I'd had in the last twelve days or more! I was tired from actually doing something, rather than just lying around. It kinda felt good, in a weird way.

The next day brought more of the same, and therapy began in earnest. After breakfast, Vinnie came to take me to the PT room for my first session. The purpose of PT was to strengthen core and arm muscles to build my ability to push myself around in a wheelchair and lift my weight to transfer from chair to bed to what-all. You know—my new normal that all the medical experts assured me would be for the rest of my life.

Because I had no feeling in the lower half of my body, Vinnie picked me up, helped me into a wheelchair, and rolled me to the PT room. The colorful surroundings, much like a kindergarten playroom decked out in primary colors, captured my attention as soon as we entered. It was stuffed to the ceiling with mats, exercise medicine balls, parallel bars, standing tables, sinks, weights, small wooden steps, stationary bikes, Hoyer lifts, and equipment designed for every possible physical handicap need. Vinnie wheeled me to a pre-set mat, lifted me from my chair, and laid me on it.

The room bustled with sound and activity that further captured my attention. I looked beyond the vibrant, sunny colors and therapy equipment to the other people in the room. Pity welled up in my stomach at the sight, and I closed my eyes in the hope I could unsee what I'd seen—a shock to my naive little world.

Children. Paralyzed from the neck down—not waist down like me. Children. With multiple sclerosis, muscular dystrophy, cerebral palsy, spinal cord injuries, brain injuries, birth defects, car accident victims with extreme injuries, and mental retardation.

A confusing mix of emotions swirled within as I watched them work with other therapists on varied types of equipment. And there I was feeling sorry for myself.

Shame on you, Paula! How dare you feel so sorry for yourself, surrounded by all these poor kids who are really suffering! Quit with your pity party, you selfish brat!

Vinnie called me to attention. "Ready to begin?"

"Uh . . . sure. Sure." My heart wasn't in it, but I engaged with the novelty of actual physical activity. It seemed like years since I'd done anything more than lie flat in my bed.

Vinnie pulled my legs out to their full extension and twisted my hips to stretch muscles that had been asleep for a while. "Does it hurt, Paula?"

"No. Can't feel a thing."

I lifted small hand weights to strengthen my arms, and Vinnie bent me from a prone to sitting position. Up. Down. Up. Down. Repeat. Repeat. Repeat. Hope sat up. Reality dropped me down. Again. Again. Again. Like an emotional rollercoaster, I felt strapped into a crazy ride. Depression sat beside me, void of encouragement. There seemed no end in sight.

However, the PT session did end, and Vinnie returned me to my room for an appointment with Doctor Nina Steg. She examined me thoroughly with optimistic remarks and a lighthearted manner. "Move your foot," she directed, as though it were the simplest thing in the world.

Move my foot? Didn't she get the memo that I'm paralyzed from the waist down? Is she in the wrong room? What kind of sadist doctor is this to ask such a stupid question to someone who clearly cannot move her foot!

"I . . . can't." *I hate saying I can't do things. Ugh!*

"Tell your brain to move your foot." She smiled and put her hand on my leg.

Well, at least I could do that much. So, I did. *Move foot, move!*

I watched her squeeze here and there on my calves and thighs. I didn't feel a thing. She looked straight and tilted her head as she moved her hand up and down both legs again. "Hmmmm," she said. "I feel a little stimulation of the muscle."

Is she just trying to be encouraging or does she really feel something? "What do you mean—muscle stimulation?"

"I can feel nerve endings twitching. Ever so slightly."

"What does that mean? Will I walk again?"

"Well, we'll see." She pulled her hands away, removed her latex gloves, and jotted notes on the clipboard at the end of my bed. "That's not something we can know at this time."

Not something we can know at this time? Then, what was that tiny spark of electricity I just felt burst up from deep within me? Depression slunk out of that seat beside me. Hope entered in an infant carrier.

"I'm hungry. When is lunch?"

"Lunch is at 12:30 p.m., in the patient cafeteria," Karen said. She was my occupational therapist. We had worked our way through another session of kindergarten classes—or so it seemed. Karen's job was to keep my fine motor skills sharp which involved many of the activities related to the education of a five-year-old.

She'd place marbles on a table, and I had to sort them by color. Then there was the shape work and writing on notepaper and other familiar early education skill building tasks to assure that no brain damage had occurred.

"Everyone eats lunch and dinner together. And if you have visitors, they're welcome, too." Karen wheeled me to the cafeteria alive with the clinking of dishes, chatter of voices, and oddly enough, hoots of laughter.

The first few days that I ate meals in the cafeteria were a little awkward. I kept to myself since I had arrived and did not venture to connect with any fellow patients. Even though I looked forward to eating—the food really was pretty good—I couldn't pull myself to interact with people.

Why do I feel so afraid of these sick kids? The cafeteria forced me to look into the faces of the other patients at the hospital and get to know them up close and personal.

35

They grouped the tables according to age, so I met other teens like me at my assigned table. But when I looked around, I saw tables with very young children. Very ill, young children.

When I allowed myself to look at them—*really* look at them—one thing stood out to me: how normal they acted. No matter their condition, they laughed and teased and seemed to really enjoy each other's company. Like a big happy family.

But they have so much to be angry about! They should really feel sorrier for themselves. They are victims, after all. It's just not fair!

I admit it. Those thoughts raced around in my mind and stirred up my own anger. About me! But from a table across the room, a flood of giggles captured my attention where a group of wheelchair-bound and braced children glowed with a level of contentment that shamed me.

Why don't I feel pity for them? I . . . I don't know what I feel.

Karen had wheeled me to a table where I met some patients nearer my age. They were in the same position I was—forced to learn a new way of life because of a physical injury.

Scott was about nineteen years old, just like me, and had been in a diving accident which left him paralyzed from the neck down.

Tommy, around our age, too, totaled a Datsun 280ZX and broke his neck. He was trussed up in a complex brace-like instrument called a halo, that looked like a jail cell mounted on his shoulders and down his back.

Jim had been beaten by his girlfriend's ex-boyfriend. His assailants shoved his head between two wrought iron railings going up a set of stairs before they snapped his neck. Trauma and injury surrounded me in such company. The four of us had lived active, normal lives prior to our misfortunes.

But Maria was different. Maria had Spina Bifida, a birth defect that happens when the spine and spinal cord do not develop correctly in the womb. An orderly rolled her large wheelchair into place at our table where she ate like the rest of us but in a reclining position. She was a beautiful fifteen-year-old whose deep blue eyes sparkled with the love of life. Maria overflowed with a sense of gratitude for every ounce of care she received. She had lived her entire life at duPont.

Think of that! Her entire life. And she's so content.

That first luncheon in the cafeteria with our little group affected me in a strange way. I wanted to be alone to think. A flurry of emotions I couldn't identify pressed upon me. Even Mom remarked about how quiet I was that evening when she and Dad and Alan visited. My thoughts were out of order, and I had no words to explain what I felt. I fell asleep seeing Maria's bright eyes and hearing the laughter of children with wisps of images from my cafeteria encounter.

Oh, God. Help! Tomorrow, more new normal and new, unsettling things I might learn about myself.

"A standing table? What's that?" I asked Vinnie when he introduced it to me at our next PT session.

"You lie down on a table, I strap you down, and it slowly lifts one end to put you in a vertical position. We do this so you don't get dizzy when you're upright."

"Upright? I can't be in an upright position." I didn't want to be argumentative, but if I'd never walk again, I'd never stand again. "My legs, you know, they don't move."

Vinnie ignored my bit of snark. "Well, eventually we'll be moving you through a series of therapies on different pieces of equipment like the parallel bars. You need to get used to being vertical before we do that."

I'd always wanted to take gymnastic lessons when I was a kid. I'd seen the cool things gymnasts did on parallel bars when I watched the summer Olympics in the past. But the bars weren't for anything so dynamic. They were only designed to strengthen my ability to hold up my weight with my arms.

"Whatever. I guess you know what you're doing." *Snark. Snark.*

"We know what we're doing, Paula. I promise you that!" Vinnie delivered his retort as though he had some insight into the Bible verse that talks about how a gentle word turns away wrath.

Back in my room, alone, thoughts of contented, laughing sick children, grateful blue eyes, and kind words spoken in response to snide remarks floated uppermost in my mind. And then—I'd see my David's face loom large before me, reaching out for me.

Visits with my family, especially David, were my reward for all the work my therapists kept me busy with—and weary in—all day, every day. I read books to him on my bed while Alan and my parents watched a TV in my room, and Dad rubbed lotion on my legs. From time to time, I caught their worried glances, concerned about what our futures might look like. For me. For them. And especially for David.

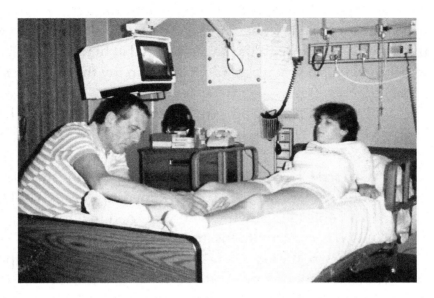

Dad, rubbing my legs and feet became a nighttime ritual. This was just like my dad to seek to always make things better for me. A generous, compassionate man who never wavered in supporting me through my trial. Even to the point of attempting to fix those things beyond his control—like his consistency to massage my legs on every visit without a word or consult with the doctors. Just selfless giving in the hopes that his efforts would help.

David was like that Hope in the infant carrier. Somehow, he strengthened me with each visit. He never looked at me any differently than before my sickness. He saw me as he'd always seen me—strong and capable and dependable with plenty of hugs and kisses to fill his heart. Plus, I still did all the silly voices in his favorite books. Bonus! He didn't see my sick condition. He saw ME. The deep down inside ME.

I needed to see ME again—the strong, capable, dependable ME, again. With my child's eyes.

"Moon. Moon." David pointed to our well-worn copy of *Goodnight Moon* on my lap and readjusted himself in the crook of my arm with his beloved Hulk Hogan action figure clutched tight to his little chest, ready for his favorite bedtime story read. I knew the words by heart and spoke them softly as he turned the pages. I stared at him in wonder and stroked his hair with a sudden lump in my throat. *I must get my life back!*

"I guess I'll see you guys tomorrow, then." I said.

Mom and Dad kissed me and gathered their things, ready to leave.

"Grrrrrr! Grrrrr!" David twirled around in the middle of the room, his face set fierce, determined to wrestle Hulk Hogan in an epic take down while Alan tried to wrestle our pint size WWF champ into his arms.

"Come on, Buddy. Time to go." Alan swept David up and whooshed him to my bedside for a goodnight kiss. I hugged them both close and hated to release them. *Thank you, God, that I can still use my arms to hug my loves.*

"Bye, Mommy. Bye!" David waved Hulk Hogan at me with one last fierce "grrrr" before he disappeared out the door flung over Alan's shoulder.

Lights out, I stared at the ceiling alone with my thoughts in the darkened room. A tear rolled out of the corner of my eye and plopped onto the pillow. I missed my husband. I missed my baby. I missed my life. I missed ME.

Could there be a Hulk Hogan deep inside, ready to rise up and power slam the villain that had pinned me to a hospital bed with a hopeless prognosis? My lids felt heavy, and my mind drifted into the twilight of slumber. That last glimpse of David, fierce with determination to wrestle his foe in an epic take down, seeded my sleep with inspiration.

With mixed resolve, I decided to begin fresh in the morning on *Operation: End This Nightmare.* I'd endure the daily doctor visits with a better attitude—even though I hated how they poked at me, over and over. *Don't complain. Don't complain.*

I'd have to work double the amount of time I was supposed to work in PT and OT. Dr. Steg said she felt something in my legs. If I worked harder, I might feel something someday—or not.

Don't despair. Don't despair. David needs me, God. Help!

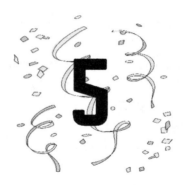

I opened my eyes at the sound of swishing water. Bright sunbeams streamed through a skylight positioned over a marble whirlpool tub where water churned and gushed in gentle swirls, crowned by a bubbly foam. A soft, lavender scented vapor rose up and flooded my being with peace and warmth. Lush greenery with exotic flowers surrounded the tub with tendrils of leaves tumbling down the three steps up into the inviting bath. I heard the flush of a toilet and looked down to see myself, seated on the proverbial throne, stark naked.

Not a soul was around. Just me. Alone.

It had been weeks since I'd been in a bathroom by myself. Joy filled my heart and I jumped up, eager to step into the tub and complete a pampering spa treatment. But, with the very hint of a step forward—I fell. Falling. Falling. Falling. Then . . .

"Paula? Paula?"

A voice from beyond called my name. With a start, my eyes flew open.

"I didn't wake you, did I?" It was Joyce. One of the new nurses who I'd just met the day before. "Time for your shower." She busied herself positioning the wheelchair by my bedside and cheerfully chattered on. "Were you dozing?"I couldn't speak.

"I'm sorry. I guess you really pushed yourself this morning in PT. Vinnie said you were a real champ!"

The dull truth of reality materialized in my understanding as I came fully conscious. I'd had that dream before—the toilet, the whirlpool spa bath, the soothing lavender scent. I didn't want to be dependent on a regiment of strangers to wait on me, wash me, move me from here to there. For the rest of my life. *Oh, God! I want that dream to come true!*

Another perky aide popped into the room. "So, are we ready?"

WE are NOT ready. I almost allowed a nasty remark to escape my lips in response until I glanced at the framed photo of David on my nightstand and remembered my new resolve. I grunted my consent to the inevitable. *Just do it! Don't complain. Don't complain.*

They wheeled me around the bed and into the cubical of a bath and shower that had no skylight, no streaming tendrils of lush foliage decor, and no warm and inviting swirls of scented lavender water. Just a handicapped shower stall with two strangers, doing for me what I dreamed to do for myself.

Push harder! Push harder! Tomorrow. Tomorrow I'll be better. TOMORROW!

The next day, I mentally put myself in gear as soon as I woke up. I had to be my own coach. Everyone around me just wanted to help me manage my status quo for the rest of my life. But I couldn't accept that prognosis. I had to push myself to go beyond expectations in everything. When the doctors dropped by with their daily visits and poked at me, over and over, I squelched my desire to grimace and groan. *Don't complain. Don't complain.*

But it was in the therapy room where I really got my game on!

DuPont used a therapy device similar to what was used in chiropractic care. Pads hooked up to a machine stimulated muscles with electrical impulses. They placed the sticky pads on my knee and turned the impulse meter up which artificially moved my knee. Like being knocked with a doctor's hammer to test reflexes, the impulses made my knee kick up due to the external muscular stimulation. I felt the hint of an electric jolt for a split second, deep inside somewhere. It was a sharp, burning sensation, just before my muscles involuntarily responded.

But if Vinnie touched me on my knee, leg, or foot with his hand, I couldn't feel it. The machine had to be well monitored because if it was set too high, it could damage my muscles.

"Try to wiggle your toes," Vinnie asked. I tried, but nothing happened.

Try harder. Try harder!

"We just want to see if we can wake up your muscles," he said.

I can do it! I can do it! I tried to convince myself.

Vinnie placed the stimulator pads all around my legs, on the back of my calves, and in front of my shins. They were placed in a particular position to make my legs move one way or another. Every time they placed the pads and turned on the machine, my toes wiggled, or my knee kicked. The therapy stimulation repeated three to four times for each area of each leg within an eight-minute time frame, per leg.

"Try this," said Vinnie, "kick your foot or lift it to the ceiling and then drop it down." I tried not to snarl at such a ridiculous request. My resolve to move on my own took the lead and attempted the impossible. Every day Vinnie asked me to wiggle and kick. I tried. And failed. Every time.

Days passed. I existed in the bubble of a routine. Nothing changed. Everything remained the same. Day in. Day out.

After two weeks, I lay in bed one morning, fighting Depression—who had fully infiltrated my room and displaced the Little Hope I'd entertained earlier. My enthusiasm for the therapy room had soured by then, so I just went through the motions, barely cordial to Vinnie when he'd arrive, cheerfully set me in my chair, and wheel me to the room for our exercises. *He's got enough jolly for the two of us.*

"Okay, Paula," he said after he'd hooked me up to pads and wires, "think and wiggle your toes."

It was a very conscious process to wiggle toes. I had to concentrate, to think hard about my toes and that I wanted to wiggle them. On purpose. I'd done this for close to fourteen days and had no reason to think today's result would be any different.

But it was!

I thought hard and tried to wiggle my toes, and—I did it. *I DID IT!*

I felt like Eliza Doolittle who finally pronounced, "the rain in Spain stays mainly on the plain," in proper English to pass muster with Professor Higgins. *By George, I got it!*

"Do it again," Vinnie said.

I did it again! And again!

My toes wiggled! Not just slight flickers of movement, but those little piggies wee-wee-wee'd wildly with a run-all-the-way-home movement. I had not been able to do that for over a month!

Tears flowed freely, like they'd been held in a reservoir and the dam broke. Vinnie called to everyone within earshot. "She wiggled her toes!" My chart said I could not do that. But there I was, up close and personal, doing the very thing they said I couldn't do. My chart would have to be changed. And so would my long-term prognosis.

Other therapists in the room rushed to surround me, patting me on the back with encouraging words. Patients unable to move from their mats cheered me on.

Crying and laughing in a rush of elated emotion I shouted, "Where's a phone! I gotta call Mom and Dad! Alan and David—your mama is coming home!"

I wanted to walk back to my room, but Vinnie wouldn't let me. *Just as well, I'd probably trip and fall for how emotional I am right now. Maybe tomorrow!*

However, after a week of overtime in the gym and therapy room, and herculean efforts at cheerful chatter in the cafeteria, and kind responses to my therapists, I saw very little results other than the toe wiggling.

I should be able to do more than just stupid toe wiggling. I worked so hard this week! Why can't I walk yet?

Depression literally kicked in the door with a keg of beer, a bakery shop of chocolate cake, and a single black balloon to start the pity party. Collapsing into a mental meltdown, I metaphorically chugged a Coors Light, shoved cake in my mouth, and determined to have an audience with my counselor, Alison.

The next day, I insisted the orderlies put me in my wheelchair. I had business to do! I boldly wheeled myself down the hall and into Alison's office. "I'm checking myself out!"

Alison shut the door behind me for privacy and spoke softly in an effort to calm me. "Good morning, Paula. What can I do for you?"

"I told you. I'm checking myself out. I don't belong here with all of these invalids."

Our eyes met for a brief pause. She sized me up to determine her next move. I wouldn't let her checkmate me. I was going home!

Then, oddly enough, she picked up the phone and moved it to where I could reach it. "Okay, there you go. Call your mother and see if she can come today to pick you up."

Ooooo. An unexpected stroke. *Is she kidding? She's not gonna try to convince me to stay?*

Alison's devious strategy was made clear as soon as I finished yelling into the phone at my mother that she should come immediately to get me.

"No! Paula," Mom replied, frantic at the thought, "you can't do that! You can't leave there yet. You're not ready. We're not ready!"

"I'm doing it! Right now! I'm sitting in this nasty wheelchair in Alison's office on her phone. She's got the paperwork ready. I hate it here!"

In reality, my wise counselor didn't have a stitch of paperwork prepared. She simply sat, pushed comfortably back in her swivel chair, and watched me make a fool of myself.

Once the conversation got heated, Alison leaned forward and provided a full stereo onslaught. She calmly tried to talk me off the ledge in one ear, while Mom lectured me over the phone in the other. Their voices rang together like wildly clanging bells in a tower and clashed with Depression's pity party raging in my head. Hope was nowhere in sight.

I dissolved into complete anarchy.

Like flashing images in my mind's eye, I saw Maria's sparkling eyes before me and heard the hollow sounds of happy cafeteria laughter. I felt mocked in my weakness, dropped the phone, and broke down in a tsunami of chaotic sobs. The violent rush of passion and emotion rushed to the surface from a place deep inside me that I didn't even know existed. I was vaguely conscious of Alison picking up the phone and saying something to my mother about how everything was going to be alright.

Allison wheeled me to my room as I emotionally shutdown, too exhausted to do anything but tremble. We passed all the kid friendly art on the walls which make me sick to my stomach. An orderly helped move me into my bed, as I gulped back silent sobs.

Alison tried to placate me with soothing words, but I would have none of it. I should be walking by now and I'm not. My world was tumbling down around me.

There, in a children's hospital, with nursery rhyme murals painted on the walls, I was one with Humpty-Dumpty. Would anyone ever be able to put me together again.

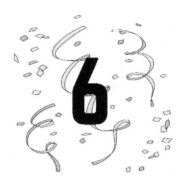

"I'll give it one more week. But if I don't see results, I'm leaving!"

Mom, Dad, Alan, Allison, and Iris, the other counselor, brought in as back-up, gathered around the bed to hear my proclamation. I'd fallen asleep after my little tirade and by the time I woke up, it appeared their troops were refreshed, and rational discourse took place. They presented their sensible science and data driven arguments while I countered with my stubborn insistence to go home. In a week.

"Okay." Allison agreed.

"We understand." Iris smiled.

"We're here for you, sweetheart." Mom and Dad assured me.

"I love you, babe." Alan stroked my hand. "You've got this!"

You bet I do! I sure told them!

Even after a complete meltdown, I still believed myself to be the victor on the field. I took full command, determined not be separated from my husband and son at the whims of bed charts, PT/OT sessions, and cafeteria meals. It was time for me to go home. DuPont served no purpose for me anymore. After all—*I wiggled my toes all by myself!*

Only one thing gave me pause to ponder: *What are they whispering about outside my room now that I dismissed them from my presence? Why are they chatting with the nurses in mysterious low tones, with frequent glances at the open door to my room?*

That afternoon, I blankly stared out the window at the play area where some of the mobile kids enjoyed the sunshine and specially designed playground equipment. I loved the rough and tumble of playgrounds when I was a kid. *Would I ever be able to take David to the playground by myself again? How would I manage it in a wheelchair?*

Susan, a new day nurse assigned to me, interrupted my daydream. She entered the room to check my vitals and chart again.

"Hi, Paula!" She toyed around with a couple of the wires and her hand knocked against the Rosary beads. Their clickity-clack sound brought a split-second vision of my mother's eyes the night she put them there and promised me that people were praying for me.

"Oh! How pretty," Susan smiled and admired the beads. "Are these yours?"

"My mom put them there to remind me of people praying." I stared off to the farthest corner of the room in the hope that she'd get the hint—*I don't want to chat.*

"Oh." She lingered for a moment and then took the Scapula in hand. "Um . . . what's this?" I twisted my neck to see what she referred to. "A Scapula. Supposedly, you can't die if you wear it." *Okay, now you can leave.*

But she didn't leave. How odd. I was suspicious of her awkward movements. They seemed staged for some reason. After all, it was too early for the vitals to be checked. They usually updated the chart later in the afternoon.

50

"Am I still alive?" A snark remark might move her along faster.

"Oh, you're alive alright."

"Just not kicking."

She smiled, though I detected a trace of pity in her eyes. I hated it when people looked at me like that, so I turned away.

As if to rescue the moment, she deflected my coldness with the most unusual request. "Can you cut my hair, Paula?"

"What?"

"My hair. I can't stand it. I mean, it's really growing out and needs a trim—if not a completely new cut. I saw something in a magazine—that feathery, mullet thing, you know? Aren't you a hairdresser or something?"

How weird! I haven't had a conversation about hair and fashion for weeks. How did the new nurse even know about me being a hairdresser? Well, almost a hairdresser.

My confused expression invited Susan to continue. "Yeah. Iris, or somebody, maybe Allison, told me you were a student in cosmetology school."

Ah. That's it! This is a counselor ploy to try to cheer me up. Get the staff to talk about stuff I like. Well, I got them on this one!

"Cut your hair?" I snapped back. "How would you like me to do that? I'm in a constant sitting position."

"Well, I can sit on the floor, and you can sit in your wheelchair. Easy-peasy."

Susan's words felt like a giant hand had reached down to a deep place inside my broken heart and lifted me out of myself to sit in a sunny spot where Hope lived. I could feel my eyes brighten, my facial features soften, and the edges of my mouth slowly curl up in a smile. Involuntary movement.

Sit on the floor? That could work. I could DO something!

In hindsight, I should have charged money, because from that moment on, I became the resident hairdresser and beauty expert. Even some of my co-patients got in on it. I enjoyed a steady stream of clients with appointments between therapies and after nursing shifts.

Nice job, counselor. You outsmarted me. I don't feel sorry for myself anymore. I feel important. Kudos to you!

Things were set in motion immediately as though it had been planned.

Alan brought my beauty school kit from home that evening. Perm rods, rollers, clippers, shears, squirt bottle, tape, combs and brushes, hair dryer, curling iron—the whole suitcase. It included three mannequin heads that I used for practice. I never named them. They were just a redhead and two brunettes and had to be relegated to remain in the suitcase. I'd have real redheads, brunettes, and even blonds to practice on. And every one of them had names.

It was awkward at first, but I quickly adapted to the limitations. My new clients were nurses, kitchen helpers, and other patients. For each appointment, they wheeled me into the rec room, designed like a comfortable little living room. My patrons sat on the rug on the floor in front of me and I'd cut their hair from the wheelchair.

I was only able to cut—no finishing with blow dry and curling irons. I couldn't use products either. Just a squirt bottle with water. No shampoo girl and no tips. Perms were impossible.

I mastered the Farah Fawcett feathered cut and the Dorothy Hamill wedge on the girls. The mullet, like Susan requested, was a favorite. I gave instructions for how to build it up into the fashionable big hair look of the 1980's disco queens with half a can of Aqua Net hair spray—like coating your locks in lacquer. Nurse Paula allowed me good practice on naturally curly hair, the hardest type to cut and manage well.

For the boys, regular guy cuts were the popular choice, some clipped short, and some longer. Although my cafeteria mate, Scott, preferred a crew cut.

I was proud to be a giver—not a taker. I made a contribution to the quality of life for those around me. The activities of my days balanced out. I poured something of myself into the needs of others, which countered the necessity for others to meet my constant needs with no avenue of equal reciprocation. I'd found a way to participate in life again! My heart settled into a place of peace, and I had happy things to share about my day when the family came to visit. David loved to see his mommy laugh again.

Though no money exchanged hands for my services, I received payment in heart and spirit from those who sat before me. Especially some of the patients. Two of them remain pressed in my memory because of the strength of spirit in their dire condition.

One little girl named Lauren, was a tiny six-year-old with severe physical limitations. She had been left on the doorstep at duPont when she was an infant—dumped by parents who never returned for her. The staff took her in, and she had lived in the hospital her whole life. It was her home. She'd never known anything else. The nurses treated her like their own child.

Lauren could hear and understand you when you spoke, but she could not talk. She only responded with a shake of her head "yes" or "no." Her beautiful features glowed with a permanent smile and bright blue eyes that looked deep into your soul. No words were necessary to mine a certain kind of wisdom from her—as from one who'd conquered suffering with contentment.

She sat in a wheelchair that reclined flat for more comfort since her condition caused her great pain. I loved to brush the thick, blond hair shafts that fell down her tiny shoulders and came up with all sorts of braids and ponytails or other styles for her—some were just silly, to make her laugh. Such a beautiful child.

Then there was twelve-year-old Teresa Marone who looked a lot like me when I was younger. She wanted a mullet cut like Nurse Susan. Teresa suffered from the same thing that bound me to a wheelchair, but she was in worse shape. Some nasty mosquito paralyzed her from the neck down. *How can such tiny creatures make life so miserable for people?*

She sat in front of me in her wheelchair which put us at about the same level. Even though she was smaller than me, I barely managed to do the job, but found creative ways to get around our awkward positioning. A flawless Mediterranean olive skin tone set off her dark brown hair and eyes to perfection. She would have grown into a striking Italian woman, but her prognosis was the same as mine—a wheelchair bound invalid life sentence.

Teresa's twin sister and parents remained constant by her side—a close family. Scott and I hung out with them sometimes in the rec room and played Scrabble and other games.

Games were like OT where we had to practice things like holding cards in our hands or picking up and moving game pieces on a board. If Teresa's sister or parents weren't there, a nurse or other patient helped her play, and we'd team up. She possessed a sharp intellect—a bright mind with engaging conversation—tragically imprisoned in a body that would never move again. Her injury occurred a few weeks before mine, so she'd been at duPont for a while and had settled into the routine of her new home. I admired how content she seemed with her lot in life, accepting her condition. I never saw her depressed or prone to complain— always thankful. *But she has so much more to endure and overcome every day than I do.*

As the official hair stylist of duPont, I enjoyed the opportunity to get to know everyone on our floor—all with similar health issues and injuries. More severe illnesses like mental retardation, lived on other floors that I did not have much interaction with.

I grew to love my new friends over the next busy days of therapy and hair styling visits. I often watched them from a distance in the cafeteria or rec room play and marveled at how they reminded me of the kids I used to go to summer camp with. Just kids, being kids, laughing together, playing together, talking about normal kid-stuff as though they didn't have a care in the world. Like Lauren and Teresa.

I learned something about myself from their humility and thankful hearts: I lacked where they were full. Suffering made them strong. They knew something I didn't know about drawing strength from catastrophic misfortune. Sometimes, craggy rocks and uneven terrain in mountain hikes don't fortify you enough for the unscalable boulders and steep stone walls in life. To conquer the mountain before me, I needed some of the intangible climbing tools my duPont friends possessed.

I had lots of time to ponder these deeper truths and search my soul for what God might teach me on this metaphorical mountain climb. My fellow patients did know a few things. I gave myself to learn from them and grow. I felt sympathy for them, awed by their resilience and the ease in which they accepted the burden of a childhood and future derailed by severe sickness.

Even so, I didn't want to be one of them. Not that I looked down upon them, but somewhere deep inside of me, I just knew—they were not my tribe, and my destiny would not be the life of a permanently handicapped invalid.

Mom tried to help me overcome what she saw as an obstacle in my mindset. "Now, Paula, I know you had your heart set on a certain future. God must have other plans for you."

"Mom, you're not helping."

"Just look at Maria or Lauren. Their situation is much worse than yours. They'll never get to go home. But you will."

"When, Mom? And what will I do when I get there?"

Mom shook her head. "Well, just a few days ago you were swearing to leave the hospital at the end of the week whether we thought you should or not."

Yep. I knew she'd throw my meltdown back in my face. And she was right. As much as I didn't want to admit it. She was right.

"Lauren has never known anything different."

"But Maria has," Mom countered. "She seems content to accept her fate."

Fate? Or faith. *If God is who He says he is, He can get me out of the hospital and make me walk again. Isn't it faith to believe that I'm justified to not accept my situation? To believe that I can get my life back and go home to Alan and David fully healed?*

I looked away from Mom and focused on the family picture of me and Alan and David taken at the Sears portrait studio that past Christmas. "I can't answer for Maria or Lauren," I said, "they have their life. Their choices. I want my life back."

That night, I lay in the dark overwhelmed with a sense of failure. A heightened awareness of my losses crushed me anew and tears flowed in an effort to flush all the ugly from my heart. *God! I don't want to fail!*

Though I couldn't feel a thing from my waist down, my condition was not my failure. What I did feel in my messy mind and broken heart was the big fail. *Gulp.* It was probably time I talked to God. No fancy prayers. Just plain talk.

The Rosary crucifix above my head reflected off a ray of light from the hallway in a golden glimmer that caught my attention. If no-fail Jesus was tough enough to willingly go to the cross and die for my fails in a horrific execution, then He was tough enough to hear plain speak from a frustrated, if not angry, nineteen-year-old wife and mother in super-fail mode—in need of some resurrection life.

I used to love sitting with God in the mountains where I learned of His love and greatness by observing all He had created—everything new every spring after the deadness of winter. Did He love me enough to create newness in me like He did in the hills and valleys in their season?

Yeah, God. You and me. We gotta talk.

In barely audible, jerky, unpolished words, I laid my heart before God and aired out my complaint until I came to the end of myself—no one to depend upon but God. I keenly felt the ugly bitterness taking root in my heart towards the family I loved, Vinnie, Allison, Iris, and all the staff at duPont. They faithfully cheered me on through the peaks and valleys of my unexpected life circumstances no matter how much snark I handed out and deserved my thankfulness—not resentment.

God and I—we made a deal after our convicting conversation that night. How much more would a humble and thankful heart, like I'd seen exampled in Maria and Lauren, strengthen me for my mountain climb? If I were to take hold of my life destiny, healed and whole again, I needed more than simple physical strength in PT to master the management of my condition. I needed an internal strength of character so that whatever destiny the Lord laid before me, I could accept in peace, resilience, and purpose. I would never be an invalid—not valid. In that, I refused to fail!

My eyelids grew heavy, and my prayer drifted into a comforting sleep. I knew—God heard me. Tomorrow would be different because I was different.

In the morning, the routine began again. A busy day of therapy and three haircuts for patients awaited me. I didn't have the inner urge to buck the system. People depended on me—I was valid!

I went into my therapies resolved to climb that mountain with a Heavenly Hiking Partner as well as my dedicated family and the duPont team. I had treated them so poorly. *God forgive me!*

With a dose of humility and shift in attitude, a fresh confidence welled up within me. Deep down inside, I knew I was just passing through, not living indefinitely, in continuous episodes of *Lifestyles of the Handicapped and Wheelchair Bound*. My life's journey would not end on that side of the mountain when the other side waited for an unfailing conqueror. I resolved to return whole to my family and all I had Hope for.

Push! Push! One more step. Just one more. You can do it! You can do it! The words I coached Donna with my last summer at camp while hiking the mountain trail on her way to victory, echoed in my mind . . .

"Two are better than one . . . and if you get God in the middle of your struggle, it's a three-fold cord that won't be easily broken."

Donna caught her breath and laughed. "You're not going to leave me. Are you?"

"Nope," I said. "And neither will God."

The mountain trail memory with Donna dissolved as Vinnie arrived to take me to therapy. I met him with a cheerful smile—not an ounce of snark in sight. Something had definitely shifted inside.

That was the day I felt pins and needles while wiggling my toes. Not electrical impulses from a machine. Pins and needles—all my own nerve endings! A little thing, perhaps, but mountains are scaled one little step up at a time.

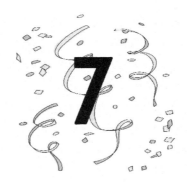

BOOM! Pins and needles in my wiggling toes! What an achievement! *Thank you, Jesus!*

CRACK! It felt like I hit a home run and points were finally put on the board for me. The doctors announced a new prognosis.

"Well, Paula," said Dr. Steg, "It looks like your nerve endings are NOT dead and we'll need to make a change in your treatment and therapy direction."

Ha! Seems like they're playing on my field now. I told them I wasn't going to settle into their invalid status quo. Just call me "No-Fail Paula!"

Dr. Steg squeezed my leg muscles to feel for nerve stimulation. "Up to this point, we concentrated on your upper body for wheelchair strength maintenance. But I think we can move more aggressively into building up your lower body strength. I have to say, I did not expect wiggling toes and pins and needles."

When the family visited that evening, we celebrated. Mom praised God, "What an answer to prayer! A miracle! An absolute miracle! A lot of people are praying for you, you know."

"Yep," Dad agreed. "It's a small step up that mountain."

Alan squeezed my hand while David sat cuddled up in the crook of my other arm growling at his Hulk Hogan doll like a pro-wrestler in a power play. "Small step?" he countered. "Hun—that's one giant leap up that mountain! Proud of you, Babe."

"Yes, but I still have so far to go!"

"What is the new therapy they talked about?" asked Mom.

I shook my head and snuggled tighter with David. "I don't know. Will find out tomorrow. It just feels so good to have a tangible hope that I can really cling to, now."

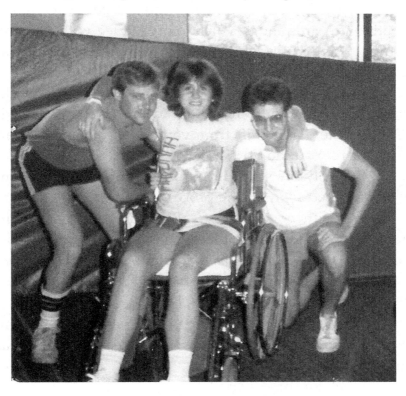

Alan and my childhood friend, Joey. We'd been playmates since the playpen. He once made me a dog food pie when we were about 7 or 8 years old. I'm wearing a seat belt. I never sat in the wheelchair without being strapped in secure.

The next day, my curiosity about new therapy treatments was quenched when we started work in earnest. Vinnie gave me a high five upon his arrival to take me to PT. "Great job, Paula! You ready for some new stuff?"

"You bet! Onward! I've got a mountain to climb!"

We began with exercises designed to build muscle on the outside of my hips. Vinnie laid me on a mat and wrapped a large rubber band around my left foot connected to my right foot. "Okay, lift and move your right leg out. Not up. Out."

This involved focused thinking to lift my leg barely an inch. Much harder than I'd anticipated. After a few repetitions of this and a switch to my left leg with the same results, I was exhausted. Undeterred, Vinnie promised more to come.

From the same position, he placed his hand flat against my foot and told me to push counter to it. "Concentrate, Paula. Lift from your hip. Your muscles are larger there. You can do it!"

But only my stress level rose—not my legs. Was my celebration too soon for the process ahead of me? I focused on lifting with a good dose of self-talk in light of my lackluster performance. *Come on, Paula—don't let your imagination run away with you. Slow and steady wins the race. You barely wiggled your toes yesterday. You lifted an inch today. What did you expect? Just keep a'going!*

Vinnie put me in a sitting position and instructed me to lift from the knee which was easier. "There! You did great! That's about a three-inch lift!"

"Yay, for three inches!"

Small muscles from the knees down seemed easier to manage and I saw greater advancement in those exercises.

Ankle wiggling ensued with gradual growth every couple of days. *Keep climbing. Keep climbing.*

I settled into a more practical outlook, sensibly concluding that even though they were little steps, at least I was going forward.

"Here's one you'll like," Vinnie said one day. "Imagine you're driving a car. You need to press the gas pedal to move forward. It's called foot rolling, to strengthen the muscle in your ankle."

"I'm on it! I get it. It's not a lot but one step up this mountain at a time and I'll get to where I'm going." *I'm determined to master this road trip.*

All the increased activity culminated in being able to stand without the standing table. Instead of strapping in my body, they strapped my legs in metal braces. The stronger material supported my weight since my muscles weren't able to do that. Yet.

"Okay, Paula," Vinnie said as he and three other therapists surrounded me. "We're going to lift and pull back. Let's see how you do."

I breathed deep and closed my eyes in a silent prayer for help. "Okay. I'm ready." With robot-like legs in those metal braces and the encouraging support of the therapists, they swung me up and into a vertical position. Then, standing. Alone!

Well—for about three seconds. Then I crumpled into their arms and therapy was over.

That night in my room when everyone visited, you'd have thought I made a triple play with all their cheers. Marianne eyes filled with tears at the news.

"It was only three seconds, Mair," I said, "Nothing to cry about."

She wiped her face. "Aren't you psyched? That's three seconds they thought you'd never be able to do! Three whole seconds, sis!"

Be thankful. Be thankful. But I admit— I struggled to be grateful for the accomplishment. Three seconds. Three inches. Yeah, it was something—but not enough.

The next day, new medications were added to my regimen. Susan brought them as I watched a Phillies game on TV. "Who's winning?" she asked.

"My guys, of course. So far it's 5 to 3 in the 6th." Mom got me into baseball when I was about ten years old. If the Phillies weren't on TV, we sat on the screened-in porch and listened to the game on radio.

Susan busied herself setting up the cup of pills on the table next to my bed. "I've brought something new today. Because you've been doing so well in therapy, Dr. Steg is starting you on steroids to build muscle."

"Steroids? Like what they're saying those baseball players are taking now?" I'd heard talk about those drugs on the news. Some of the professional ball players took them to build muscle. But in 1986, it was still too early before the steroid controversy became a scandal.

"Yeah. It should help you improve in PT."

My arms had grown firm and strong through therapy. I worked hard to build up what still worked. Every day I sweated through exercises to help me better push my body up and out of my wheelchair; to move from bed to chair, chair to mat, wheelchair to shower, and what-all. In fact, I'd lost a lot of weight with all that upper body exercising. When my PT focus extended to my lower body, the doctors felt I needed a little extra juice to "up my game."

How cool! I'm on the same regimen as professional baseball players for performance enhancement!

Enhancement nothing!

"They think this stuff will help my muscles recover, but the only thing it's doing is making my face break out," I whined to Alan after a couple of days on the new meds. I inspected my appearance in a hand mirror. "Ugh! I gotta deal with this now, too."

"Well, be thankful you're not still looking like the green alien—the way you did right after this thing started." He laughed, then tendered looked into my pock-marked face. "You're still beautiful to me."

I winced with split second conviction that I'd slipped into a pity party attitude again. But as I lifted the mirror to study a particularly offensive patch of acne on the tip of my nose, I snapped out of my good intentions and complained. "Well, from my point of view, this stinks."

Alan tried to change the subject. "Did the Phillies win today?"

I nodded, turned to look out the window at the fading sunlight, and lost myself in random thought.

The Phillies did win and had been winning more games than normal. They started out with average stats but forged ahead with a burst of energy to push them into some great wins around the time I hit the hospital, about two-thirds into the season. I had a lot of hope they'd make it to the playoffs and maybe even win the series. No matter how disappointing their performance was early in the season, I tuned into every game believing for the win and ultimate victory by season's end.

As darkness fell on another long day at duPont, it dawned upon me that I was living a baseball season of my own. And it wasn't over til it was over. The wins would come. Some might be glorious with a blowout and multiple homers. Some might be clinching it in the 9th. A slump over a week or two of games was inevitable. Rising from a slump was, too.

My life felt like a baseball game. Triple plays and home runs in one inning. Foul balls that deceive the eye to where you think you got a hit only to find it's just taking you one step closer to an out. Ups and downs. Ups and downs.

I never wavered in my belief that after a loss the next game would be a winner. I was a loyal Phillies fan. I needed to be that kind of loyal fan for myself! I drifted off to sleep later that night thinking on these things and resolved to decline the invitation to my pity party, get on the field in the morning, and own home plate!

The next day started with a bit of a win when one of the nurses arrived with welcome news. "We're going to remove your permanent catheter today, Paula!"

I was giddy with joy. I hated that nasty catheter. It got in the way during PT and was just plain ugly and annoying. Because I had no feeling in my bladder, I didn't know when I had to pee. Prior to my new prognosis, the permanent catheter seemed the logical approach. But now that I needed more freedom to exercise my lower body in PT, the staff came up with a new plan to help me pee.

"One of us will come to catheterize you every 2 hours or so," she said. "No more of those nasty bags you don't like."

"Oh," I said. Then the force of the plan hit me like a foul ball. How humiliating! *Talk about losing your modesty — every two hours, every day?*

It was awful to have people fuss about in my personal area so often, but I got used to it after a while and it became just another part of my daily normal. I was thankful for an abundance of female nurses available to do the job and dreaded the very thought of a male nurse doing it.

I felt pretty good about myself with so many hits and runs early that week, until I looked in the mirror at the end of the week. That one annoying patch on my nose had multiplied everywhere. Within a handful of days, gross lumps and bumps and red rash eruptions marred my porcelain, beauty queen complexion.

Marianne visited towards the end of that week and could not conceal her shock at my appearance. I burst into tears, knowing why her eyes bugged out and mouth contorted in horror. She quickly recovered, put on her big sister shoulder pads for me to cry on, and promised a solution.

"How will anyone in the hospital take me seriously as the resident beauty expert when I look like this!" I sobbed.

Marianne was a champ. She let me blubber all over her. "Don't you worry, hun," she said. "I know just the thing! I'll make a special trip back here tomorrow and you'll see. No worries, now."

True to her word, she did return the next day with an arsenal of acne medicated facial cleansers and creams. I eagerly used them with great hope in their effectiveness. Truthfully, the outbreak was only a temporary side effect of the steroids and lasted a couple of weeks with no scars to stain my pride and joy skin. But, while in full zit glory, I obsessed over the blemishes with constant magnification mirror inspections.

"Pool time!" Vinnie enthusiastically announced as he entered my room. "That should cheer you. A new addition to your PT routine."

I tossed the mirror onto my nightstand and pretended that I hadn't really been laboring over my facial distortions. He pretended he didn't notice.

"Pool? I can swim?"

"Well, not exactly. But, well . . . you'll like it. It'll help you in more ways than one."

Hmmm. More ways than one. What did he mean by that? They mentioned pool time would be added and I had worked out in my mind what it would be all about. *It might help heal my acne if I splash enough chlorine water on my face.*

I had pool plans! I was an expert swimmer. I could do laps. I could dive. I remembered my summer camp days not long ago, spending a lot of time in the Olympic sized pool with my friends.

More recently, David, at 2 years old, had learned to swim from the time he learned to crawl. We did mother/child classes at the YMCA so he would be water safe. I loved splashing about with my dear baby boy. He'd jump into the deep end of the pool, and I'd catch him. And we took full advantage at Alan's mom's house where they had a pool for summer fun and exercise.

Yep! I had some real plans for pool time.

However, once Vinnie delivered me to poolside, all my big expectations went *POOF*. The therapists had other ideas. What a disappointment to realize that my pool dreams--much like my spa tub dreams—were just that. Dreams.

Pool time was regimented work, not play time. They strapped me to a pool chair Hoyer lift and lowered me into the water where a nurse moved my legs up and down. Invalid pool time. My hopes to lift my spirits in the pool melted away with my self-esteem.

Windows at the top of the high ceiling allowed sunlight to drift into the room, but there wasn't any sunlight that day. In fact, storm clouds had rolled in and raindrops bespeckled the glass panes as they emptied like tears from dark clouds that blocked blue skies.

Up. Down. Up. Down.

The somber atmosphere outside and repetitive manipulation of my lifeless legs by the nurses lulled me into a melancholy reverie, counting my losses. I was a very healthy young woman. A high school basketball player, roller-skater, hiker at camp, one day—and the next—all gone. A life stripped away. Paralyzed. Living far from my husband and precious little boy whom I loved so much.

David needed a Wonder Woman mommy and here I was, being manipulated around in a pool by two nurses as if I was a bendable action figure doll with no ability to act or move on her own without a puppet master operating my limbs in clumsy motions.

A rush of heavy wind and violent beat of rain on the windows arrested my attention upward to see the clouds darken the sky like dusk at mid-day. My thoughts grew dark, too.

Is this it, Lord? Is this what I have to look forward to in life? The living dead? Maybe I should just be dead. I'd be less trouble for my family when I get home. If ever I get home. Their lives will be turned upside down, if I do . . . caring for a zombie invalid instead of the vibrant wife, mother, and daughter I used to be.

Pitty-pat. Pitty-pat. The rain outside echoed as it beat against the window glass.

Pity-party. Pity-party. The rain in my heart followed suit as it flooded me with discouragement.

I didn't feel like doing much the rest of that day. The black clouds outside followed me inside to my room after pool time. I shutdown and slumped as the nurses cheerfully prattered on, dressed me like a Barbie doll, and settled me in my bed. Part of my new night garments before sealing me under the covers involved moon-man boots. Or so they appeared to me. I guess I was astronaut Barbie!

Apparently, when the ankle muscles begin to move after paralysis, they must be kept in special boot shoes while sleeping so the toes are pointing straight up to the ceiling. This flexed posture guards against the ankles relaxing the foot into a dropped position—foot drop. This would not allow the muscle to heal normally.

Thus, I was trussed up to wait out the hours til nighttime. Would I have that recurring dream again of a courtroom where I pled my case before God, to no avail?

"I don't belong here, God. There's been a mistake! The doctors are wrong. I know they are. Send me somewhere else where they will know how to fix me."

Silence from the bench.

"Why me? What did I do to deserve this? Didn't I spend every summer at Christian camp and help all those kids? Wasn't I a great coach for Donna that day in the mountains? She praised me and said she couldn't have scaled that mountain without me. Don't I get points for that?"

Deafening silence from the bench.

"I'm broken. BROKEN! God! Fix me. Fix me, please?"

The dream always seemed to end about there. Still no sound from the bench—but a sensation. I felt His smile. He and I had had this kind of conversation before. Many times.

Thank you for being so patient with me, God. Maybe I need to be patient with me, too.

Awake in the morning, I felt horrible inside, conscious of the ugly thoughts and emotions that had surged through me in the dark of night. All alone.

"Give me something to smile about today, Lord."

The morning sunshine filtered through the curtains, freshly drawn by the orderly who brought my breakfast. The storm passed. Blue skies and hope for the new day dawned on my heart. My eyes drifted to another picture of David on my dresser. He was hugging his Hulk Hogan doll and had a stern look of determination on his little face to mimic his wrestling hero.

I smiled. "Thank you, Lord. Thank you."

It's amazing what a touch of gratitude can do for your psyche. I playfully grimaced my best Wonder Woman searing-with-determination face at the picture of David. *I'm on it! New day—let's play! Thank you, Jesus!*

I crushed it at PT. Astounded the natives in OT. And imagined I was a mermaid princess being fawned over by her team of attentive servant codfish at pool time.

When I returned to my room, that black cloud knocked on the door seeking an encore visit. I was bored, tired from all the activity, and felt a bit low. I didn't have anything to do which left me vulnerable to pity parties. The Phillies weren't on. No hair appointments that day.

I absentmindedly toyed with my hands and realized they needed a makeover. *Something to do! I'll give myself a manicure in my favorite hot pink nail color and shoo that nasty dark cloud away.*

Nurse Amy came into the room to catheterize me and stopped to admire my manicure when it was complete. "Oooo. That's pretty! What's it called?"

"Not Really a Waitress."

"What?"

"True story," I laughed. "Not Really a Waitress. That's what it's called." I motioned to my nightstand where the nail polish bottle sat.

Amy picked it up to inspect the name herself. "Hilarious! Who gets paid to name nail polishes so crazy like that?"

"I don't know. But it's been around forever." I held my hand out in front of me and we both admired the manicure. "Regardless of the name, it always makes me happy when I wear it."

"Well," said Amy, as she fluffed my pillow behind me, "It's good to see you smile. That makes ME happy."

I was touched by her personal attention, and we proceeded to chat about random things. The hospital shifted to shut down, nighttime mode, so she had a few minutes to visit. We talked about our families and discovered we both had a weird obsession with Ralph Macchio from *The Karate Kid*. It was fun to just kick back—so to speak—with girl talk about things that had nothing to do with hospitals or Hoyer lifts.

"Speaking of Ralph Macchio," she said, "don't you think Scott looks like him in the eyes kinda?"

Scott was the 19-year-old boy in the room next to mine. He had been in a diving accident which paralyzed him from the neck down. We'd shared some good laughs in the rec room playing cards and cafeteria over meals, but I'd never thought he looked much like Ralph Macchio. I didn't see it.

"Oh well," Amy sighed. "Guess it's just me." She looked at my hands again, then slowly raised her face to gaze directly into my eyes. A mischievous grin widened across her face.

What on earth was she thinking?

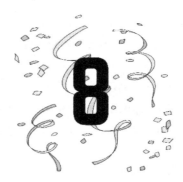

"Shhhh! Stop giggling!" Amy stealthily wheeled me out the door and into the hall.

I pursed my lips and muffled my adrenaline rush of excitement. "Quiet! I'm quiet." I didn't want to mess up our well laid midnight plans for mayhem. The most fun I'd had in weeks was the anticipation of Nurse Amy's brilliant idea for a little levity.

When Amy saw that I had nail polish, she thought it would be a great prank to sneak into Scott's room and paint his toenails in the middle of the night. His room was next to mine. We shared a wall between us.

The short trip for making a bit of mischief while the residents slept reminded me of camp capers in the dead of night that I played on unsuspecting campers during my summers at Sandy Cove. We thought up some whoppers, back in the day. We put people's hands in a bowl of water while they slept which prompted them to pee the bed. The stealing of clothes in the night hours elicited screams of panic in the morning when campers had nothing to wear. And the popular toilet paper cabin wrap made the 8-person habitation look more like a mummified mausoleum forcing helter-skelter cleanup before morning inspections.

Though not as messy or complicated, Amy and I completed our operation with muffled giggles in a timely manner. With mission accomplished, we crept out of his room as silently as we'd entered and left Scott with a professional nail job in Fire Engine Red. I snickered myself to sleep that night, with images of how he might react when he woke up and realized he'd been pedicured!

His response did not disappoint.

"Paula!"

My eyes popped open at the sound of my name bellowed from the other side of the wall.

"Paula! Get in here and get this #&%@* off my toes!"

It took me a couple of minutes to collect my thoughts before I remembered my midnight foray into misconduct. I burst out with a gusty guffaw and one of those uncontrollable snorts as if a pressure plug exploded from deep within me. It felt great!

Poor Scott! Boy, was he mad at me—not a happy camper. Still, he provided choice entertainment to the patients and staff on the floor in his pranked distress. Too bad my cohort in crime, Nurse Amy, had left at the end of her shift and missed the fireworks.

I laughed all through the removal process. His searing glare, like curses, pierced me through as he impatiently waited for me to finish. I wondered if we'd ever be Scrabble buddies again. Or maybe, the next time we played, he'd have a few choice words to share on the board in my direction.

But at lunch that day, we broke bread together in peace and he admitted he could see the humor in it all. Good on him. Retelling the story gave everyone else at the table, who'd missed the show in the morning, a good laugh, too.

We all need to loosen up and laugh at ourselves once in a while. It breaks up the stress of taking ourselves too seriously—especially when we face grim life challenges.

After so much stimulation and adventure, I returned to my room hungry for more. *Who can I prank on now? Tomorrow? The next day? Nurses? Patients?*

Clever thoughts of who and how to prank consumed me over the next couple of hours but ended in nothing resolved to the purpose. I'd be dependent on others to assist me in my machinations and didn't think I could get anyone to partner with me in a regular course of mischief.

That's when Vinnie popped his head in my doorway. "Hey! Wanna go bowling?"

"Bowling! From a wheelchair?" I asked, shocked at the bizarre invitation.

"Sure. Doc put it on your PT list as a new activity."

"But, how? Where?" I peppered Vinnie with enthusiastic questions as I eagerly moved from bed to wheelchair. Prankster dreams faded at the prospect of this inviting turn of events.

Vinnie wheeled me out of the room and into an elevator. He pushed the button for the basement of the hospital—a place I'd never been to before. Once we emerged from the lift, we turned right, and the hallway opened into a real, live bowling alley!

I felt like I was in some sort of time travel tunnel going from my hospital room to the Fun Zone Alley back home. I half expected to see my friends Russ and Kris and Joe and Dina and the whole old gang that Alan and I hung out with. We didn't bowl in a league, but regularly met at the Fun Zone before David came along. Our routine was always the same: settle into our assigned alley, grab greasy food from the concession stand, and team up for a night of good times and laughter.

I fancied myself quite a bowling diva with a high score of 220. I used a 10-pound ball and threw right-handed. "Your turn, Paula!" Dina would say. "We can take these guys!'

I'd smirk at the taunts of our male opponents and step to my place on the starting mark. "This is how it's done, boys!" I lifted the ball and moved into my windup: short left step, short right step, short left step, right behind left foot, right arm behind back, right leg up, next to left foot, and right arm release of the ball down the alley with a graceful glide skyward, my thumb pointing the way in one fluid sweep. STRIKE!

"Another strike!" Joe cried, shaking his head in disbelief. I'd thrown three in a row and was pretty proud of the accomplishment.

"WhooHoo!" I ran to Dina and jumped up and down to celebrate then skipped over to my fries and Coke for a victory gulp. "And it's all your fault, Joe."

"My fault?"

"Sure! You're the one who taught me that little thumb trick. You know—when you bring your thumb up straight it steers the ball to roll straight and hit the target. I've been practicing!"

Joe rolled his eyes and got a fair ribbing from the rest of the guys for giving his bowling secrets away. It was all in fun since the bunch of us bowled at the same skill level—no handicaps necessary.

"So, what do you think?" Vinnie's voice snapped me back through that time tunnel, simultaneous with the sound of a ball hitting its target.

"Huh? Huh? Think?" I blinked myself into my present reality—wheelchair bound with three therapists surrounding me. A bowling alley in the basement of a hospital.

My heart sank. There I was—former bowling champ with a LIFE handicap. Oh, for just a little more time in that time tunnel!

Even so, my confidence rose, and a rush of determination welled up from deep within me. I refused to allow a total of four therapists spotting me to steal this adventure. I had to make the most of it!

"Give me that ball!" I demanded.

Vinnie handed me a 10-pound ball as another therapist wheeled me to the line. No step, step, step for me this time. I was instructed to turn the chair a quarter to the right and swing my arm back, then forward to release.

I followed through with the toss and my arm's muscle memory kicked in with a graceful sweep upward, my thumb pointing to the sky, just like Joe taught me years ago. The ball rolled down the lane slower than I'd been used to, but it eventually reached its destination. No gutter ball! In fact, my heart leaped at the sight of one by one, a handful of pins bobbled and fell at the end of the lane. Not all of them, I admit. I wasn't quite my old bowling diva self. But— some of those pins fell to the sound of enthusiastic cheers from everyone.

Victory WAS possible. One pin at a time.

Victory WAS possible. One challenge at a time

I'd faced the challenge of those pins and continued to watch them fall with every straight shot of passion and effort I threw into it. And the ball. Thumbs up to the sky in a confident, graceful swing, each time.

More cheers that evening, back in my room, when Alan and my parents arrived for their visit. I told them how I improved with each throw, managing both the chair and the ball like a pro. "And Vinnie said that when you guys visit sometime, you can go down and bowl with me, too."

Alan and I reminded each other of more bowling stories with our friends and I caught a glimpse of Mom and Dad watching us. Mom's eyes glistened with emotion. Seeing me expressing joy encouraged them.

I liked how it felt to be an encouragement to someone else even though my own situation was less than perfect.

That week was eventful beyond the midnight prank and bowling triumph when the doctors fitted me with crutches for the first time. My muscles had barely begun to work again, and my legs remained weak and wobbly. The doctors assured me that I would never be able to walk unassisted.

On the other hand, my arms had grown muscular and strong due to all the therapy work which enhanced my ability to master the use of my new Canadian crutches. These were metal sticks with cuffs that wrapped around the upper arms with a handle I grabbed onto with my fists. It gave me more stability than wooden crutches and distributed most of the weight on the crutch rather than on my legs.

It felt great to stand upright again. I didn't need a round table of therapists holding me up and the more I worked with the crutches, the less likely I was to crumple into their arms.

Towards the end of the week, as I rested in bed gloating over my triumphs, I felt a painful pressure in my lower abdomen. I hadn't felt anything there in weeks!

I didn't want to jump to conclusions. Or panic because of where I felt the pain and pressure. A less rational mind might jump to worst case scenarios: *I have a tumor!!! My bowels have dissected!!! I'm pregnant!!!*

I shut my eyes at such nonsense and simply rang for the nurse. To my relief, Nurse Amy responded. "Problem, Paula?"

"Amy!" I pointed to where it felt strange. "I have this odd sensation about here. A kinda pain—or pressure."

"Okay." She nodded her head, calmly walked to the supply cabinet, and pulled out a catheter.

"It's not time for that."

"Well," she winked, "it just might be."

I allowed her to position the catheter and within seconds a great rush of fluid exited my body. The pressure released to my great relief. And elation!

"See," she said, "you felt that you needed to pee. Congratulations!"

My smile must have been a mile wide. "I felt the need to pee!"

"You felt the need to pee." She grinned and dislodged the catheter.

"I felt the need to pee!"

"Yes, you did."

I felt the urge to jump out of bed and victory dance, but my muscles refused to cooperate. So, I did the next best thing. I shouted at the top of my lungs, "I FELT THE NEED TO PEEEEEE!"

Amy burst out laughing and our unbridled celebration brought another nurse, an orderly, and Dr. Steg into the room to see what all the noise was about. Once they arrived, we accelerated into full blown party mode. And it was no pity party, either. My progress turned a corner that day. It was my first full week of winning and I liked winning. I wanted more winning.

Dr. Steg asked me a couple of technical questions and scribbled some things on my chart.

"Do I get to go home now, Doc?" I asked.

"No, no. Not yet."

No, not yet. But soon. I just knew I'd be going home soon. *And when I get home, I'm going home able to pee, to wiggle my toes, and with Canadian crutches rather than as an immovable invalid in a wheelchair.*

When the family arrived that night, we continued our celebration with more pee talk than when David started potty training. I basked in greater HOPE than ever as I drifted off to sleep that night. Surely, I am Wonder Woman and will be home soon with Alan and David—and using the bathroom by myself for the bonus win!

My faith grew leaps and bounds that week, even though the milestone did not deliver me fully from the need to be catheterized. The 2-hour pee schedule, whether I needed it or not, was no longer necessary. I'd tell the nurses when it was time for catheterization instead of them telling me. I felt powerful and in control.

But my excitement was short lived, and faith tested, when jubilation was replaced by mortification around lunchtime the next day.

I had to pee and pressed the nurse button for assistance. Brian, the only male nurse on the floor, came into my room and pushed the nurse light off. "What can I do for you, Paula?"

"Um . . . I need to pee. Is Amy or one of the girls available?"

"Well, I'm the only one here. Everyone else is at lunch. Can you wait a little?"

I lowered my eyes and mumbled, "Not really."

My bladder nerves were not normal yet, so when I did feel the sensation to pee, it was very strong. In fact, it burned. I needed to be catheterized immediately, but the thought of Brian, the male nurse, performing the job flustered me.

Brian sensed my uneasiness. "I can help you. Is that okay?"

My acne had started to fade, but in that moment, I felt it multiply and grow beet red all over my face. I never wanted to have to pee again. I just nodded and looked out the window, refusing to make eye contact with him as he emptied my bladder. The last ounce of modesty I had left vanished.

When he exited the room, a melancholy spirit descended upon me. All my big wins that week shattered to the ground like so many cheap trophies fallen from a high perch. My pee win turned out to be a loser after all since I couldn't really control the management of it. There was no guarantee that a female nurse would be able to assist me and every chance that Brian would be the only help available to me in the future.

The future.

Okay, God, I guess I should thank You that I can pee, but now I hate it. How embarrassing to have Brian stick that tube in my privates. He's just a couple years older than me. Ugh! I hate that I'm so dependent on others for daily needs. I hate that I can't do things by myself. So what if I can feel that I have to pee or that I can wiggle my toes or stand with crutches or bowl or go in the pool, even. Big deal! I can't do any of it on my own without one or more nursemaids to make it happen. And what an idiot I am to think I'm gonna go home anytime soon. I'll have to take an army of nurses and servants home with me to get me through the day. I'm no Wonder Woman. What kind of life do I think I'm gonna have as a mother to David? Or a wife to Alan?

I turned away from the sunlight and blue sky shining through the window at midday and buried my face in my pillow, conscious of tears spilling from tired eyes. Broken in body and spirit, my faith, buoyed by a few big wins that week, turned out to be a bust. I failed.

Or I thought I failed.

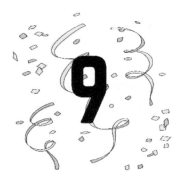

"Come on, Aunti-Pau, let's take a ride!"

I felt a tug at my arm that drew my attention away from an evening chat with my sister Susan. She and her husband John regularly visited me along with Marianne and Dean.

Susan was a stay-at-home mom to April, my sweet five-year-old, blue-eyed, blonde haired niece. They lived in Northeast Philadelphia, but when they visited, David delighted in his feisty cousin as a playmate.

April's tiny fists gripped my sleeve and yanked on my tee-shirt with importunity. "Come on! Come on!" Her relentless pleas enticed David to follow her lead. How could I resist their petitions?

"A ride! A ride! Let's go for a ride!" I laughed and turned the wheels of the chair out the door, followed by two munchkins who jumped and clapped and giggled with glee in anticipation of what they called a "ride."

In fact, only I went for a ride while they pushed the wheelchair up and down the hallways, laughing hysterically the whole time. I added muscle to their kid-power since they couldn't shove the chair hard enough. My buff arms provided the brawn to make the wheels go round for great fun. Often, we'd wheel over to the rec room where our visit continued. This was the same open living room space where

I gave my free haircuts and beauty treatments to the staff and clients and played Scrabble and cards with my fellow patients.

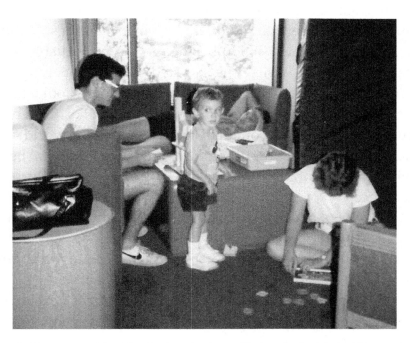

I took this picture of David enjoying playtime with Joey in the chair, Alan on the sofa, and my best friend Kris working a puzzle for David on the floor of the rec room. It was a bit clinical in hospital furniture design, but it was the closest we could enjoy to our own living room at home.

But to April and David, it was the playroom— the main reason for wanting to take me for a ride. They had romping room to twirl about, and the grownups sat comfortably on multiple couches and chairs of the industrial, hospital variety. April and David forgot all about me once we arrived there and made way for the primary-colored rugs and toys—a more welcome sight to visiting toddlers and preschoolers than my stuffy hospital room.

On the frequent visits with David and April, we spent a lot of time in the rec room playing games, working puzzles, and reading books. I wanted to make David's life as normal as possible so playtime with Mommy was important. Teenage Mutant Ninja Turtles often accompanied David if Hulk Hogan was unavailable that day. On April's visits, she assisted him in the guise of Wonder Woman to save the world as Susan and I looked on.

How I wished I could sit on the floor like April and be David's Wonder Woman instead. I'd make the world safe from mosquitoes that put innocent mothers in hospital beds with threats of an unjust, life-long, wheelchair prison sentence.

When possible, we ate meals together. David and April craved ice cream for dessert from the soft serve machine. The chocolate and vanilla twist was a favorite, and they embellished their treat with rainbow sprinkles.

I loved the sound of their giggles. There is nothing so healing as the melody of carefree children laughing. *Oh, to be a child again!*

Though neither of the kids remember much about that season of our lives today—as I write this account decades later—at the time they were much involved in my recovery without them even knowing it. I drew my resolve and determination to heal from them. Each visit was a booster pill to my resilience and perseverance to walk again. To return to normal living. For them.

I always slept better after a visit with the kids, nodding off with a smile on my face. Tomorrow would bring new challenges, but David and April fortified me for my fight.

One morning, after an especially joyful evening visit with my little loves, Vinnie entered the room with a big smile on his face.

"Well, you look happy today. Have a date last night?" I teased.

"I am happy," he said. "Look what Doc put on your chart!" He held out my chart and pointed to something scribbled on my PT to-do list: "Parallel Bars."

"Parallel bars. You mean like gymnastics?"

"Not quite," he said, holding my arm as I pushed myself into my chair. "We're gonna work on you standing between the bars."

Pool time. Bowling. Now parallel bars.

At the first mention of it, I had visions of Mary Lou Retton taking the 1984 Olympics by storm with her gold medal performances. *That'll be me! I've got the arm muscles for lifting my body and flinging it about, for sure.*

I remember watching Retton's routine on the uneven bars which included a move that came to be called, "The Retton Flip." She transitioned from a front flip, low to high-bar, and ended up sitting perched on top of the high bar. A "ta-da" moment for sure and worth the gold she won.

As we entered the PT room and wheeled up to the bars, I resolved to have my own gold medal win moment to boast of to David and April. I had quite an obstacle to overcome. Paralysis. Just to stand between the bars would be a win to be proud of. But I wanted more.

Vinnie and I chatted about Mary Lou Retton, and he told me how she had to overcome a lot to earn her gold. She was born with hip dysplasia—the ball and socket joint of her hip had not formed properly. Years of competitive gymnastics aggravated the condition. Even so, she powered through any pain, discomfort, or adjustments she experienced to achieve great success in front of the whole world.

My whole world was David and Alan and my family. As Vinnie lifted me to place my hands on the bars—left and right—I thought of them and tossed aside my Wonder Woman aspirations to settle for Mary Lou Retton, Olympic Gold Medalist level goals. *I don't even need a gold medal or an Olympic dream. I just want to walk again!*

Conquering the parallel bars was not an easy feat. Even with some of the recent improvements I'd had with leg movements, I still had zero strength in them. My arms held up my entire body while my legs hung lifeless in a vertical position. The therapists cheered.

"Fantastic, Paula!"

"Look at you go, girl!"

"Paula! We are so proud of you!"

I nodded along with a weak smile in response to their enthusiastic encouragement. "So, this is good?"

Another round of cheers and even a pat on the back ensued.

"Okay." I shook my head and looked down at the two lumps of legs below, just hanging there. "I guess you know what's good. If you're glad. I'm glad."

In truth, I was discouraged.

They did most of the work that first day on the bars. But unlike Mary Lou's spotter who supported her in flips and twirls and leaps, my therapists just moved my legs from the ankle and pushed them forward one at a time without bending my knees, as though I were walking. I tried not to feel disappointed.

My arms were solid and strong enough to well support my weight. I should have gone into competitive arm wrestling with my build. Perhaps the Olympic wrestling team? Each day I'd found it easier to transfer myself—by myself—from bed to chair and back again due to my upper body strengthening.

When we returned to my room after the discouragement of the first bars day, I playfully slapped Vinnie on his wrist when he tried to lift me. "Nope! I want to do this. Let me move myself from the chair to the bed." I flexed biceps and triceps and scrunched my face in determination.

He laughed and backed away, "You got this, champ!"

I closed my eyes and imagined I was Mary Lou Retton about to flip herself onto that high bar and land with all authority like a Queen on her throne. The Queen of gymnastics. *Just let me be the Queen of flipping from my chair to my bed, Lord.*

Deep breath. Push. Launch! In one power thrust, I was airborne and landed on the fluff of the side of my bed with only the hint of awkwardness. Vinnie spotted me and helped the rest of the way. "You did it, Paula!"

"I did it! I did it! All by myself!" High fives and whoop-whoops filled the room in celebration of the milestone. "Mary Lou Retton, eat your heart out!"

Word got out of my grand accomplishment for the day and varied staff members peeked in that afternoon with congratulations. I felt showered with gold medals because of their response which seemed to outdo the toe wiggling celebration.

Over the next couple of days, I did more on my own, and my confidence skyrocketed. I grew more independent and felt so alive that some days I thought I could jump out of bed, stand up straight, and walk right out of my room.

Realistically, I couldn't. But every day I improved, and my hope meter rose to the next level.

The end of June rolled around as the days swiftly passed. I had spent a full month in duPont. July 4th was just around the corner.

I loved Independence Day weekend. We always had a big barbeque and pool party—complete with a volleyball net in the water. Alan and I lived with my in-laws, and they had a big built-in pool and patio that required many parties throughout the year—and always on the 4th of July.

The men played horseshoes while the women, family and friends, sat poolside in bathing suits with tall glasses of iced tea and lemonade. We watched over the kids in their swimmies and gossiped. Throughout the day we filled up on plenty of summertime menu favorites: burgers, dogs, potato salad, baked beans, watermelon, and all manner of pies and sweets.

Once the skies darkened at dusk and the pool was secured, we threw on jeans and tee-shirts and headed over to the football field at the local high school to watch the fireworks. This year would have been the first year we'd take David to see them. I was concerned that he might be squeamish about the noise and the big booms, but I had other things to be concerned about that year. Like not seeing any fireworks at all—let alone spending the day with my family.

"How are you feeling today, Paula." Dr. Steg entered the room and woke me from my daydream.

"I feel pretty good. Ready to run a marathon, at least."

"Really." She gazed through my chart and marked a couple of things on it. "That's good to hear." There was an awkward pause before she raised her head, looked me square in the eye, and asked, "Do you think you might feel up to a trip home?"

Did I hear wrong? Surely, Doc didn't say the words I've only dreamed of for the past six weeks. "Home?"

"Well, it's the 4th of July weekend. Do you think you're strong enough for a little home visit?"

My mind raced wildly as I blurted out, "Yes! YES! I feel fantastic! I'm ready! When do I leave?" No way would I even hint that I might not feel ready to leave my 24-hour care. I wanted to go home so bad.

"It's just for a couple of days, Paula, but based on your progress, the staff and therapists agree that you're secure enough to go home for Independence Day weekend. We can stabilize you and see how you respond."

"Really?" I thought I might be dreaming and pinched my arm. "Nope! I'm awake and you really did say what you just said! Independence Day!" I shouted it loud and clear.

And as much as I love my country and saw myself as a patriot, I didn't mean America's independence. It was MY Independence Day. Even if it was just for a weekend.

"You know, Alan has been preparing things for you."

"He has?" I thought about flowers on the table. Perhaps some presents. A cake? *Yes. A party in preparation of my homecoming would be just the thing.*

"Yes," Dr. Steg continued, "we gave him the particulars about a handicap ramp and how to move the furniture around to best accommodate your chair and a few other things, like . . ."

I stopped listening at that point. I wanted the flowers and the cake. I wasn't interested in my home being completely redecorated in my absence—for a handicapped invalid.

" . . . so how does that sound? Paula? Paula? You listening?" Dr. Steg looked at me with a note of concern.

"Oh! Uh . . . yes. I heard you. Yes. I'm good. I want to go home. Thank you so much."

That was as gracious as I could muster with the flood of thoughts and emotions that swirled within me. My stomach fluttered with butterfly nerves mixed in a bubbling froth of anticipation and the strange desire to jump for joy and crumple into a puddle of tears all at the same time. But I kept my keen head and just smiled as Doc left the room. And me—alone with my raging thoughts.

This would be the first time I had been home since the middle of May when my nightmare began. The next morning, I eagerly prepared for the trip and couldn't stop smiling when Alan walked into the room to get my bags. He left to pack them in the car and Vinnie wheeled me down the hall, into the elevator, and out the front door of duPont to where Alan waited.

"Your carriage awaits, milady!" Alan put on a silly English accent and bowed with a flourish of his hand as he held the car door open. I fought back tears when I saw that white Ford Escort hatchback. It wasn't the dreamy metallic blue T-bird I'd always wanted, but that little bare-bones car never looked so good.

Once secured in the passenger seat, I felt like everything was new and fresh and old and familiar all at the same time. "You ready for this, babe?" Alan asked as he put the car in gear.

"So ready! Let's go home!" We pulled away from the curb and I waved at Vinnie and Nurse Amy who had escorted me out. That's when the tears welled up beyond flood stage and the dam burst into a fury of emotion as I sobbed for joy.

Joy! And just a little anxiety about what obstacles I might face in the next 48 hours of my long-awaited independence.

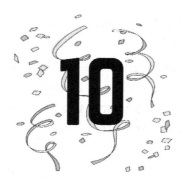

That first weekend home overwhelmed me with both joy and discouragement—a reality check that would set me on the path of either determination or defeat.

The 40-minute drive time flew by. I pointed out all the familiar landmarks as if I'd never seen them before and breathed deep the bay water air as we sped across the Delaware Memorial Twin Bridges into New Jersey. *Home! I'm going home!*

"Oh! That giant cowboy! I love him!" My giddiness was unfettered. "And look! Cow statues!"

Alan grinned and shook his head as we passed the sprawling Cowtown Rodeo grounds on Route 40 and their long-time signage attractions.

"Oh look! Corn fields!" I soaked in the view—acres of green stalks reaching to the sun in good old Woodstown, New Jersey.

I'd seen these things a million times but as we passed them that day I felt as though I'd seen them for the first time ever.

Soon we rounded the corner to the long stone driveway lined in cedars and oaks and maples, resplendent in full foliage. I wanted to stop the car and hug the mailbox as we entered, but Alan continued driving.

Mom's impatiens, in shades of purple, fuchsia, and white, encircled the base of each tree along the way. "Oh look! Flowers!" I giddy giggled with delight and Alan laughed along with me.

Of course, there were flowers! There were always flowers. As a consummate gardener, Mom took great pains each year to make the property a showplace. But that day, it was as though I'd never seen it before. Everything looked so glorious and new. I had a sudden, fresh appreciation for even the most mundane aspect of the yard.

"Hostas! Look at the hostas lining the walkway, Alan!"

"I know, hun. They've been there for years."

"I get that," I tried not to sound defensive. "But it always looked like weeds to me before. It's all so beautiful! So green and leafy." I paused in childlike wonder, feeling every inch like Sleeping Beauty just awakened after a one-hundred-year slumber. "They weren't there the last time I was here," I mumbled under my breath as I absorbed the beauty—the portulaca, hydrangeas, ivy, blooming azaleas, rhododendrons.

And—the ramp. *THE RAMP?*

Reality smacked me in the face. Yes. The ramp. That nifty preparation thingy that Alan had worked on for me—according to Dr. Steg.

"We're here!" said Alan. "And all ready for my girl to come home." He motioned at the ramp and smiled proudly.

I nodded with a sigh as he got out of the car and walked to the trunk to extract my wheelchair. It took him a minute or so to open it and put the brake on before placing it near the car door.

"Let me help you," he said as he opened the door and positioned the chair.

"No!" I put my hand up sharply. "I will do it myself."

Alan backed away but held the chair still as he watched me awkwardly finagle myself out of the car and into the chair using my arms. In that moment I remembered a recent session in PT when Vinnie included a bucket seat exercise—moving from faux car seat to wheelchair. He had prepared me for that very moment.

A rush of people flew out the front door to greet me, all talking at the same time. Mom's smile beamed with joy as she bear-hugged me before I even made it to the ramp. Tears welled in Dad's eyes as he reached for my hand and kissed my forehead. Alan's parents bubbled over with euphoric greetings and David tried to climb onto my lap screeching my name over and over. I helped him snuggle into the chair with me.

"Dinner's ready!"

"Comfort food, dear! Spaghetti and meatballs!"

"Did you remember the garlic bread?"

"Ice cream!"

Chatter about food and drink swirled around me as I tried to process my swirl of emotions. I was not prepared for how I felt. Or didn't feel—like I was disconnected from myself and watching a movie play out. Overwhelmed, I gulped back an involuntary sob in my throat and worked to fight back tears.

Why do we swallow emotion in critical moments when we should want to hold onto and cherish them rather than suppress them? My heart was full and chaotic. No PT or OT prepared me for what swelled within my soul and queasy stomach. To move forward, I shut down all the feels and just went through the motions in silence and absorbed everything like a precious gift to process later. I had no words.

Crossing the threshold into the living room, nothing had changed since a few weeks ago—though it felt different and new. The mix of paneled and eggshell brown plaster walls surrounding appointments of orange, gold, and avocado green floral velour furniture on a rust-colored shag carpet never looked so inviting.

But, when I saw the rain lamp, then I knew I was home!

You remember rain lamps—a bit gaudy by today's minimalist or farmhouse decorator standards, but all the rage in the 70s.

Imagine a Grecian goddess in a classic pose standing on a round disk platform of plastic greenery with a canopy light over her head. Three thin poles connected the top light to the bottom disk with a series of clear, twisty nylon strings woven up and down, surrounding the solitary maiden like prison bars. When the light switched on, a small motor in the bottom pumped mineral oil up the straw-like poles to gently drip to the bottom again, hugging the nylon string as tiny beads of oil. It mimicked glittering raindrops with mesmerizing movement. Suspended from the ceiling, it appeared magical and elegant back in the day. An optical illusion of a surreal world.

Being home after weeks in a hospital felt surreal to me. At duPont, I was like that Greek goddess, solitary in a prison behind bars that held me captive. But that Independence Day weekend, I'd breached the bars of my rain lamp, and nothing felt quite the norm from what I'd known of the past few weeks. Even so, I didn't miss my hospital room platform of plastic faux leaves one bit.

Dinner around the table must have been the second half of that strange movie I both watched and starred in at the same time. It seemed to be in another language though. Things I'd done all my life, in that instant, felt foreign. Was I really there? Maybe I was just dreaming. Surreal again.

Mom's choice on serving spaghetti, however, was spot on. I'd eaten it a zillion times, but that evening felt like the first time ever and I enjoyed every bite while taking in all the laughter and conversation at the table. Home, sweet home.

"Paula looks tired." Mom's brows furrowed at me with concern. "You ready for bed, dear?"

She was right. A couple hours after dinner full of carbs and my favorite sweets, I really was wasted from all the excitement of the day. I looked forward to sleeping in my own bed. But being home, even those few hours, I realized how different living life as a handicapped person would be—especially in my own home.

My bedroom was a welcome sight, but my bed at home was not adjustable like my bed at duPont. Hospital beds were nifty creations that lifted and supported the back in a sitting position. I missed that little perk when it wasn't there to help me handle the unpleasant task of inserting a catheter in my privates with a mirror for reference. I recently mastered that feat, a necessary task before they would allow me a holiday on my own.

In my bed at home, managing the mirror and catheter without the back support to do the dirty deed, made things not only difficult but more loathsome than ever.

Getting comfortable to fall asleep was a whole other story. I had no way to easily adjust my feet or reposition my body in a bed that only allowed me to lie flat.

Eventually, though, I drifted off to sleep thinking about my momentous day and focused on that Greek goddess imprisoned in her surreal rain lamp world. As I lay, less than comfortable in my own bed, I realized I'd taken my surreal world of duPont with me. They told me it would always be with me. Home would never be real for me again.

Stop it, Paula! Don't go there! I chastened my heart—or maybe it was God's still, small voice speaking to arrest my attention toward the blessings I had that were real. After all, I was home with my loves.

Sudden gratitude welled within me. I was determined to make the best of a bad—even of a bed—situation and slept soundly until dawn.

Morning arrived with new mountains to climb. After waking, I transferred myself from bed to wheelchair and decided to make the bed myself.

My mother-in-law, Dot, tapped at the partially ajar door as I settled in the chair and picked up a handful of blue floral sheets. I had just separated them from the matching spread, ready to put into real world practice what I'd been taught in OT. *You've got this, Paula-girl. You've been training for this moment for weeks! Going for the gold in bed-making from wheelchairs—a new Olympic sport!*

"Paula," Dot's charitable voice smacked me, in the moment, with a touch of condescension. "Let me do it. You can't manage it."

What? I can't manage to make a bed? Ouch!

I bit my tongue and curtailed a smart comeback to what felt like an insult. "Thanks, but I can do it. I NEED to do it." *If I'm going to be in this chair for the rest of my life, I must learn how to function from it by myself.* I smiled and turned back to the business at hand, cutting her off from further interference. She got the hint and gave me my independence but remained in the room as supervisor.

Once the last smooth was made on the bed and I turned to the door where she stood, the expression of surprise on her face made me glow with pride. *Showoff!*

"Now," I said, "How about some breakfast!"

We arrived at the table spread with cereal and juice to fortify us for a busy day. Then back to my room for washing and dressing and a bit of primping to look spectacular for my first public appearance in weeks. Alan dressed David which gave me extra time for glamour prep. It felt good to look good. Wheelchair notwithstanding.

By mid-morning we were on our way to downtown Elmer for our small-town 4th of July parade. It was nothing to attract TV cameras—just traditional Americana celebrating Independence Day in our own way. Kids decorated their bikes with red, white, and blue streamers, proud to cycle down Main Street alongside fire trucks with honking horns, hooting sirens, and swirling red lights. The high school marching band and color guard performed patriotic tunes with beating drums and trumpets that made my ears ring as it stirred my heart.

Misty tears of pride and hope surfaced as I remembered the price paid for our freedom and independence at the sight of the American Legion members who marched past carrying Old Glory—the highlight of the parade. As a grand finale, a lone trumpeter played the National Anthem. We sang along as the whole town gathered, some with their hand on their heart, some in salute.

What a beautiful sight—everyone standing to honor flag and country.

Everyone—except me.

Tears welled again in my eyes, but this time it wasn't due to patriotic fervor. I shed tears of frustration and anger because I couldn't stand on my own two feet to honor the flag like everyone else. Like I'd done for years at Independence Day parades.

Oh, God! Will I ever be independent again?

Thankfully, there was so much going on around me that I masked my red eyes and choked my emotions enough that no one noticed. Soon the band broke ranks, the fire trucks zoomed back to the fire hall, and cyclists pedaled to their parents on the sidelines as the crowd dispersed, everyone to their own festivities at home.

We arrived back at the house where Mom and Dot had stayed behind to set up a picnic feast on outdoor patio tables. It was all ready for us and I almost wanted to cry again at the sight of it. It had been too long since I'd eaten anything except for hospital food and the occasional treat brought in the evening by visitors.

But what a bounty lay before me on the table now! Squeezed together in display on the red and white checked tablecloth were an abundance of salads, burgers, hotdogs, sweet Jersey corn on the cob, watermelon, summer fruits, and an assortment of blueberry, apple, and cherry pies! *Do I have room in my stomach to eat it all? Yes! Every bit of it!*

It seemed everyone I knew was in our backyard that day and treated me like a guest of honor. *A guest? In my own home?*

Normally, we always hosted a crowd of people at such events, but this time I saw folks I'd not seen in years—and some I didn't know. But we welcomed all, and like Jesus blessing the loaves and fishes, we never ran out of food or hospitality.

It was quite a party. To some degree, the jollity of the day devolved into something of a forced pity party. Well-meaning people created awkward and sometimes downright embarrassing moments when they tried to talk to me. They didn't know what to say and I struggled to know how to respond when I'd hear things like, "How do you feel?"

How do I feel? I mean, how do I even begin to answer that? Hey—how much time do you have?

"So, what are you going to do?"

Oh, I don't know. Sign up for the next Boston Marathon?

"Can you still finish beauty school?"

Can you still finish kindergarten with a stupid question like that?

"Will you still be able to take care of David?"

No. I'm putting him up for adoption.

"Is it really hard to go to the bathroom?"

Are you kidding me? Want to know the gory details?

Each attempt to say something that might encourage me turned sour, like so much annoying noise. You know, that "whaugh, whaugh, whaugh" that Charlie Brown's teacher always sounds like? And then Charlie Brown slinks off into a corner somewhere for a pity party? Yeah, that. He doesn't even get angry first. Just deflated.

I admit it—I censored for snark my initial response to each dumb question. I felt cornered, like Charlie Brown. But not of my own volition. I didn't want a pity party, but it was being foisted on me.

STOP THE PITY PARTY!

I wanted to scream after a bit but held my growing anger. However, when Sandy, a random friend of a friend, tried to be thoughtful and consoling, I lost it. She bent down to me, like I was a five-year-old who'd put my shoes on the wrong feet, and said, "So, Paula, do you think you'll ever be normal again like us?"

No words. I had no words.

In fact, I did have words, but David was on my lap at the time, and I drew blood when I bit my lip from a critical vocal response to such an insulting question. *Twilight Zone! I'm in the Twilight Zone with mindless, heartless zombies! This chick ain't getting anything out of me.*

I winced, let David down to run off an play, then thrust my right wheel around to spin away from her and speed to poolside for a little respite. Escape from senseless idiots that assailed me beyond my patience meter with their so-called concern for my well-being and future, occupied to much of my time that afternoon.

But poolside didn't provide shelter from the storm as I watched everyone splash and laugh and canon-ball into the deep end while I sat sidelined. Instead of twirling around the shallow end with David in his swimmies, I could only observe, physically disconnected from the action.

Alan brought me another hotdog, and I bit into it with a vengeance. It scared me a bit to sense my anger meter rising to levels I'd not known before. Not even in the hospital. Being home and unable to live as I'd always lived stirred emotions in me that I didn't understand. My fists clenched.

Is this what the rest of my life will look like? I am dead to everything I'd always dreamed of if this is all I have to look forward to.

Tears threatened my eyes again, and I excused myself as I took the last bite of the hotdog, leaving a clump of mustard on the edge of my mouth. I insinuated my need for a napkin and headed to the table in a swift exit from the scene. In truth, I wheeled myself to the front of the house, out of everyone's sight, and let the waterworks flow.

Resentment and rage touched down on my heart like that mosquito again with a mouth-syringe full of pity, ready to inject its poison into the depth of my being to finish the job it started back in May. That scared me more than anything. Giving into pity meant that I gave up, and to give up after all the progress I'd made threatened to steal any future advancements. Then, for certain, hope for my life — and as a mother to David — would be shattered.

That dark, emotional moment stirred a fresh resolve to fight against a forfeit to pity and its dismal aftermath. In my mind's eye, I saw that monster mosquito with his poison syringe at the ready and flinched in a fierce response of determination. My resolve catapulted to firm decision. I believe God gave me eagle's wings to lift above the abyss of surrender and swat that mosquito and pity pumper away from my heart. Surreal again, in such a setting, I fought a battle in the matrix of my being.

I will not live like this, God! I don't accept it for my life, for my marriage, for my David, for my future! I WILL overcome this curse! I refuse to fail!

When I cried out to God at duPont, I noticed that within a day or so I always made progress in something that surprised everyone. What the doctors said couldn't be done, I did, and knew God had something to do with that.

Me and God—together. We did it before. We'd do it again. After all, what's the point of praying if we don't expect God to answer our prayers? I think that is what faith is all about. Nothing super complex. Just—believe. I had to believe. Any other option was untenable to me.

"That's it!" I spoke aloud my prayer to Heaven. "God, when I get back to duPont, I'm going to be in control. WE'RE going to be in control. Independent me—dependent on You—and in control of my own destiny!" Ugly sobs poured forth again and I shouted as loud as I could, "I will be set free!"

The ringing of my own voice made me aware of my surroundings and, in a sense, woke me from a bad dream. A comforting quiet embraced me, invaded only by the happy sounds of merry-making voices on the other side of the house, splashing in the pool. I heard birdsong with honeybees buzzing nearby and wheeled closer to study them among the azaleas in the front garden. I watched them in awe. In silence. And peace flooded my being. I traded my tears for laughter—the best exchange of goods ever.

That 4th of July in the summer of '86 was, in a way, my OWN Independence Day. No longer would I be oppressed by a physical handicap. No longer would I allow that mosquito to have power over me. I felt like my condition was a microcosm of our nation's plight in 1776—oppressed under the dictatorship of a physical constraint. I would never take for granted the idea of being free, at liberty, and independent in my body as well as my heart and mind.

But as our War of Independence reminds us each year we celebrate it—freedom isn't free. It must be fiercely contended for.

Whatever I have to do. Whatever it takes. I will walk again!

My father-in-law rustled the rhododendron bush as he rounded the corner of the house and interrupted my solitude. He had noticed me from a distance in the front yard and walked over to check on me. "You okay, Paula?"

I brushed my eyes clear, but he saw. Red swollen eyes after ugly tears always give you away.

He picked an azalea sprig from a nearby bush and handed it to me. "You know something, Paula, you can do anything you set your mind to."

I loved my in-laws, Dot and Al Aron. Dot helped me with David, looking after him, during the day while I was at beauty school and Alan was at work. Al was good to us, too. He had a big heart and I think a few secrets from the years he served our country in Vietnam. He knew a thing or too, but never let on how wise he really was—except in choice moments.

That day, when he met me in the front yard, was one of those moments. He repeated his powerful words, "Paula, you can do anything you put your mind to."

He understood battlefield faith. You don't get through combat without it. I will never forget his words as I sensed them from God's lips to my heart. An answer to prayer for direction—with great hope.

I will not give up. I will walk again!

Later that evening, after everyone left and the family crashed together in the living room, exhausted, I caught my mother staring at me. "What? Why are you looking at me like that?"

"Paula, you have a head like a rock."

What on earth does she mean by that? I glanced over at the rain lamp and that poor gal stuck inside her plastic optical illusion prison. I refused to be her.

"Thanks, Mom. You always know what to say." I tried to curb the sarcasm in my delivery. She meant well. Everyone meant well. They feared I wasn't accepting reality. But sometimes, reality is what you make of it.

Al came to the rescue—another choice moment of wise words. "Well, Ann, having a head hard as a rock isn't always such a bad thing." He winked at me and redeemed my mom's ill-conceived remark. "It'll be an uphill battle. It'll be tough going. But with your hard head bound and determined—you can do whatever you set your mind to, Paula."

I knew Mom didn't approve. But Al was out of the room before she could counter with her idea of a reality check. She saw my face, resolute and strengthened. Sometimes all we need is one ally in the fight to change surreality to reality. It all depends on how you define your terms.

Like Jacob wrestling with the angel and demanding, "I'm not letting you go until you bless me," I resolved to wrestle with what lay ahead and not give way in this life to a stinkin' disability. Time to squash the mosquito and live blessed.

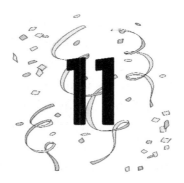

"Okay, Vinnie, I have made up my mind. I absolutely refuse to spend the rest of my life in a wheelchair. So, whatever we have to do, let's do it."

Vinnie looked at me in shock. He had just arrived in my room for our first PT since my return from home. He paused a moment before he spoke, and something sparkled in his eye. A knowing glint. Like he had a secret. "Oh. So, I guess you had a great time this weekend."

"I had . . . a come to Jesus' moment this weekend."

"A what?" I don't think he expected that response.

"You know. A do-or-die moment when I made a decision. A life changing decision."

"And what did you decide?" He shook his head like he already knew the answer.

I smiled, moved my legs over the side of the bed to position for a transfer to my wheelchair and announced, "I'm going to walk out of this hospital."

Vinnie held the chair as I settled myself in it like a pro. "Well then, Champ—let's do this thing! I've been waiting for you to get your game on!"

With my new attitude adjustment, PT was actually fun instead of tedious. It's amazing how a change in perspective can alter everything about you and your world. Back to the mats and steps and pedal-pushers and parallel bars and pool exercises I went with Rocky Balboa's eye of the tiger. I could not be stopped.

Dr. Steg and Nurse Amy watched me with great interest. All the therapists, nurses, doctors, and counselors noticed the difference in me, too.

"It's great to see you throw yourself into your therapy, Paula. What did they put in the hot dogs and corn-on-the-cob you ate when you went home for the 4th of July?" Dr. Steg said as she reviewed my charts with numbers rising to meet each new goal above and beyond expectation.

Amy was especially proud of my progress. "You know, kid, you used to be a real downer before. But look at you now!"

"Yeah. How did you even stand me just a couple weeks ago?"

"Well, I tried to distract you with your hair clients and midnight pranking. But it looks like we don't need that anymore."

"Oh, no! I don't plan to give that up. I'm always ready for some midnight escapades. I got some new nail polish I'm sure Scott will just love!" We dissolved into laughter and brainstormed a bit of possible mischief. Amy wasn't just a nurse. She had become my friend. I would miss her when I left.

And I would leave—sooner rather than later if I had my way about it. I could see a finish line on the horizon and was bound and determined to get to it running, not wheeling.

This new leaf I'd turned over appeared to inspire more than just my medical team. Maria cheered me on my way like that Olympic champion I envisioned myself to be.

Many of the other kids helped me celebrate my successes daily with encouraging words.

But poor Scott. I don't know if he still held the Fire Engine Red nail polish fiasco against me or not, but he rarely had a good word for my efforts.

In the cafeteria, where we'd meet daily with everyone, I'd share my new accomplishments. Everyone congratulated me except him. He lay there, paralyzed from the neck down, and wouldn't say a word. I'd catch a glimpse of him out of the corner of my eye and feel his scorn.

Then, I felt pity.

For him.

It was a terrible sensation. He was so helpless in body, mind, and spirit. I never wanted anyone to look upon me with the kind of pity I suddenly felt towards him.

When we played Scrabble together, we met on a level playing field and got along well. We enjoyed each other's company as friends. But as I advanced in strength and restored skills, with new milestones met and finish lines crossed, he distanced himself from me as though we were strangers. I tried not to feel like I had to please him, but a part of me wanted his approval. He, for whatever reason, could not give me that level of acceptance.

Maybe there is some truth to the old adage, "Misery loves company." With each win I attained, he saw the commonplaces that we shared in our health circumstances erode. It was selfish of him to want me to remain as much a prisoner to my wheelchair and condition as he was to his bed and a lifetime of paralysis. *If my injuries were as severe as his, would I refuse to take joy in my friend's progress?*

My new habit of soul searching led me to not pity him but empathize with him. And forgive him. For my own wellbeing, I accepted his lack of support in my goals and achievements and moved on.

As I sat in the cafeteria with everyone, I turned from the lonely Scott to the others and noticed Miranda looking at me oddly. She was about seven years old, paralyzed from the waist down due to a gunshot wound. Her father was a police officer and she decided to play with his gun. There appeared to be hope that she would make a good recovery one day and her young age helped with her happy attitude.

"Why are you looking at me like that, Miranda. Oops! Do I have ketchup on my face?" I had been enjoying a cheeseburger.

"No," she said, and scrutinized my face intently.

"What? What? You're freaking me out?"

"But," she said, "You have something weird growing on the side of your nose."

Ugh! I did. And on the side of my left cheek. And the bottom of my chin. And a large landscape making its way across my forehead. A fresh acne outbreak due to my steroid medications.

Dr. Steg insisted a stronger dose of steroids was necessary to help build muscle. "Well Paula, you know there is a possibility that the nerve damage is too advanced for you to walk, but we'll work as hard as we can to help you reach your goals."

I appreciated how the staff worked with me to help me reach my goal to walk again, but the tradeoff involved more intense therapy sessions and meds that made me break out and gain weight. If I wanted to get my legs back, I had to be willing to gain a few pounds and have a few pimples — and expose myself to a seven-year-old kid bringing attention to my facial disfigurement in front of everyone over lunch.

My good friend Kris and her fiancé Russ visited often—at least twice a week. We played Scrabble in the rec room or played with David and chatted about wedding plans, the music they should pick, problems booking a photographer, what to serve at the reception, making wedding favors, and the like. I loved having something normal and wonderful to look forward to.

Our discussions proved motivational towards my recovery. She asked me to be her maid of honor and I desperately wanted to walk down the aisle the following year for my bestie. *I must walk again!*

Kris' color theme was a scrumptious silvery-blue. We poured over the pages of dress ideas in bridal magazines to find the perfect style for the wedding party and I imagined how I'd look in each gown. I longed to feel the flow of silky skirts against my legs as I walked in a pair of elegant high heels like a supermodel gliding down the aisle. Perfect hair. Perfect nails. Perfect makeup. And maybe even a trendy picture hat!

After all those weeks in the hospital, hanging out in shorts and tee shirts, I craved a little elegance in my life for a change. A wedding would be just the affair for it.

But with every dreamy thought, as we brainstormed wedding details, I battled the nagging voices of Doom and Gloom with attempts to crush my hopes for Kris' special day.

Doubt grew louder, too, with taunts and terrors in my mind at the turn of each page in the magazines. *Oh sure, be in the wedding—in your wheelchair, pal! Won't matter what you wear. No one will see it all tucked into your invalid—in valid— chair. You'll probably get your wheels stuck on the carpet and rip it on the way down the aisle. Everyone will look at you with pity and you'll steal attention away from the bride because you're soooo needy.*

I closed my eyes to shut the noise in my head out. *I will walk! I will walk! I will dance at Kris' wedding!*

"Paula . . . Paula . . . " Kris noticed my momentary distress. "You okay?" She reached over and touched my hand.

I held her fingers tight and opened my eyes. "YES!" I spoke a bit louder than necessary. "What time is it?"

"Um . . ." She pulled her hand away and looked at the watch on her wrist. "It's a quarter to three. Why?"

I smiled and shook my head to rid the negative thoughts from further assaults. "I have another PT session at 3 o'clock. I'm working overtime so nothing'll keep me from walking down the aisle and dancing at your wedding!" My eyes teared up and I noticed her eyes slightly welled, too. Neither of us were willing to let loose the waterworks.

"I'm sure Vinnie will be in soon, then, to get you. I should go."

"No. I'm responsible for getting myself to PT now. It's part of taking ownership of my recovery mandate."

"What's that? Part of the process here?"

"Part of MY process. I made it up. I decided to be more proactive and take more initiative in my healing. I'm more aware of schedules now. Always checking on the time. I do not want to be late for PT and OT."

Kris looked at me with the same expression resolve I saw in her eyes when we determined we'd beat the boys with a high score at bowling. "Then, you'll need this!" She removed the trendy new Swatch Watch in a shimmery pink jelly strap that she'd picked out the last time we went to the mall. *She loves that watch! Why is she slipping it around my wrist?*

"No. No, Kris," I protested. "I can't take your watch. You just got it. I have a clock on the wall here."

"Well, you'll need it if you're in the common room or somewhere else without a clock. Take it."

I looked down at the watch on my arm and stroked the soft jelly strap.

"Really. It's my contribution to help you in your cause! Now you'll always know what time it is."

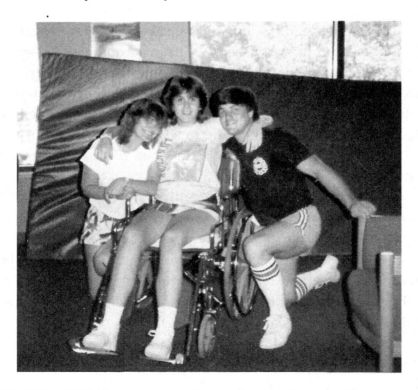

July 1986---Still, to this day, my best friends, Kris and Russ, were there for me the whole time through my ordeal. David called them, Aunt Kit and Uncle Rutt. Notice I'm wearing the Swatch watch Kris gave me and she's sporting a new one as a replacement. What a special gift that was to encourage me to always be on time for my expanded PT regimen.

"And I'll always think of you."

Cue the slightly awkward pause before a spontaneous bestie hug. She swiftly gathered up the bride magazines and was out the door just in time for me to get to PT. I pushed myself extra hard that day.

Later in the evening my parents, Alan, and David arrived as they did every night. Dad rubbed my legs and feet as usual, like it was his assignment or something. I'm not sure why. Maybe he thought it would help to stimulate and circulate blood through them. He quietly did his duty while Mom prattled on with all the news from home and made sure I was brought up on everyone's doings.

Marianne's wedding—yes, more wedding planning—occupied most of the conversation. Mair's wedding came before Kris's wedding, and I was in both. I needed to be walking and dancing again by fall. Was that a realistic expectation? The nagging, negative voices, chattering in my ears again, threatened to consume me with their shrieks. I clenched my eyes shut to quench them.

Thankfully, no one noticed my momentary panic, and Mom changed the subject to David's exploits at home at play with the kids she looked after.

Wedding woes receded to the back of my mind as she distracted me with the scene of little girls playing with their Barbies. "And then, David wanted to play, like a good sport, with the Barbie games. Well, of course the one thing all little girls want is a Hulk Hogan action figure crashing their little fashionista party. David, show Mommy how you and Hulk Hogan helped the little girls play Barbie today."

David made a fierce face and swished Hulk Hogan in the air with his arm, "Grrrrr! Grrrr!"

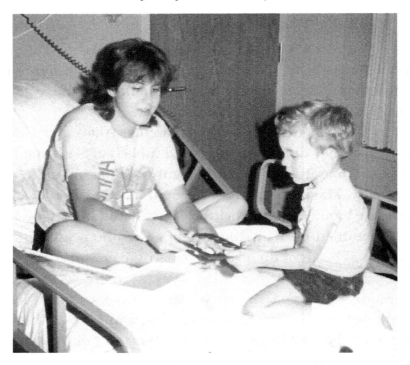

Playing with David on my bed—like two peas in a pod—I'd fold my legs into Indian style with my hands. It felt sort of normal, not all laid out like half a corpse in a bed. I wore the Scapula around my neck in this picture. It has an image of the Archangel Michael and a blessing attached to it that whoever wears it is protected from death.

I laughed to know how he tortured the sweet Barbies with his menacing Hulk. Mom said the house filled with squealing little ladies until she called them all for snacks and a VHS movie.

David continued to exhibit his best Hogan impressions, and I felt a twinge in my stomach. That sick, empty sense of loss. How I wished I had been there watching him—and not my mom.

Someday. Someday soon. I. Will. Be!

The evening visit continued much the same as every evening. Alan sat on the edge of the bed channel switching the TV in search of a game. David shared a snack with me and cuddles. Sometimes we read the books he brought in his backpack or worked on a puzzle together.

After they left that night and I readied for bed, my conversations about wedding plans in regard to Kris and Mair occupied my mind. I daydreamed about the bridesmaid and maid of honor dress shoes I was supposed to wear, which made me think of my closet at home. And my shoes there. My pretty shoes. I missed them.

Just then, Paula, my older nurse, came into the room and as if she were reading my mind said, "How about we fit you for a nice new pair of boots!"

"Boots? What do you mean?"

She pulled out a pair of nasty astronaut boots and smiled, "Tada!"

"But those are foot drop boots. I get a new pair? I thought I was getting something more stylish."

"You don't want your feet falling. Your muscles haven't worked in a while and these boots keep them flexed up." She tucked my feet into the boots and strapped them into position. "There now. They may not be the height of fashion, but they are sensible shoes to the purpose. Once you gain your muscles back your feet will work properly you can wear all the fashion boots you want. And you'll thank me."

She left the room and turned down the light. I lay in bed with her words repeating through my mind. My lids grew heavy. Sleep seemed imminent when the force of the last thing she said shocked me wide awake with revelation.

"Once I get my muscles back!" I spoke aloud. "I'll wear fashion boots again? Lord, that sounds like she knows something. She KNOWS! I'm not crazy to believe I will walk again. I am getting stronger and better every day. And

Nurse Paula knows it! She knows it—and maybe the doctors do, too!"

I prayed—my voice rose with excitement. I didn't care who might hear me, either. "Thank you, Lord, for another encouraging day. I love my friends and family. I love my new watch from Kris—God bless her! I love my new boots and I will sleep well tonight. No negative nag voices! Tomorrow will be a productive day in PT, I just know it. Oh, God! I have so much to live my best life for. Help me, Lord—to be best and walk again!"

I was all set. I had a new watch and new kickers and new resolve for a full recovery.

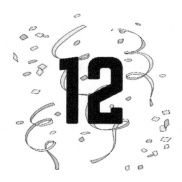

Since my triumphant return to duPont after that momentous first weekend home, my transformation astounded the doctors and staff. I swiftly advanced to new perks in treatment and therapy—not the least of which was regular weekend visits home.

Weekdays I focused on recovery with a vision ever before me of walking out of that hospital to never return. I dreamed about it day and night and felt empowered by the goal as I noted daily improvement.

Weekend home visits stirred me to hunger more for my goals achieved to their fullest. Though the tedious packing and unpacking required extra from everyone involved, I enjoyed the new challenges, and my family couldn't do enough for me.

Alan, Russ, and Kris picked me up one Friday afternoon for the drive home and we took a side trip to the Christiana Mall as a treat. I loved shopping and looked forward to the familiar echoes of footsteps and voices in the mall corridors. I was ready to take in all the luscious smells of the food court and planned to order the greasiest burger with every imaginable topping. *Oh! I hope there's an Orange Julius there, too! I haven't had that frothy dream-sickle drink in weeks!*

Frustrated at how slow they wheeled me out of the hospital, I almost took charge, but tempered my eagerness to be on the road. However, when they wheeled me to the car, I did take charge!

"Okay, you guys—stand aside! I've got this! I can arm wrestle every one of you with my buffness from PT workouts. You betcha I can manage getting into a car by myself."

"Whoa! You got this, hun!" Alan put his hands up in submission to my will and backed away grinning. Was he laughing at me or just beaming with pride at his capable wife?

"You go, girl!" Kris cheered me on.

I positioned myself between the door and the seat and pushed up on the arms of the chair like I'd practiced with Vinnie. But this wasn't PT, and I had a new audience to impress.

Perhaps it was my zeal to do so that made me try to sweep into the car like a dancer leaping gracefully from one mark to the next. Sadly, as I shifted my rear to put it onto the car seat, my attempt couldn't have been further from a ballerina's grand jeté. In a series of jerky moves I missed the seat entirely and . . . SPLAT!

A mix of alarm and laughter filled the air as my audience rushed the stage to my side. A flurry of arms and giggles tried to lift me off the ground, but the hilarity of the situation did not dissipate easily. In fact, all three of them thought it hysterical to leave me on the ground in all my inept glory.

My butt on the blacktop, I felt the palms of my hands gritty with dirt and pebbles, as I'd pushed against the ground in a failed effort to break my fall. I wiped them against each other to clean the debris and waited until my husband and best friends got their fill of entertainment at my expense.

"You finished?" The laughter died down to snickers, then silence. They knew I was peeved and swiftly readjusted their facial expressions to one of concern for my wellbeing. Kris asked the pertinent questions to determine that I was no worse for wear while Alan and Russ tried valiantly to not burst out into another round of guffaws.

"Here. We'll help." They spoke in unison and lifted my arms and limp legs to deliver me squarely onto the seat of the car.

Once in the car and belted in place, I wondered what had gone so wrong. I'd done that maneuver a zillion times in both PT and OT. We sped onto the highway as I rehearsed it all in my head again and realized where I failed.

I failed.

None of us put the brakes on the wheelchair. But they were not at fault. I was careless to shoo them away, intent on doing it all by myself with a show-off attitude. That, coupled with my eagerness for our trip to the mall and then home, made me look like a circus clown in the middle of a slapstick comedy routine.

Yeah. Show-off!

My physical abilities were useless if I allowed emotion to override important details. Things I always did before without thinking, like walking and jumping into cars, required a step-by-step protocol when bound to a wheelchair.

From that moment on, I made it a habit to check the brake every time I got in and out of my chair so it wouldn't roll backwards or land me on my bum again.

Once we got to the mall, we sought out the Orange Julius. With my first sip of their trademark drink, all my clown-show regrets melted away and I thoroughly enjoyed every minute of my Get-Out-Of-Jail card weekend.

Over many weekend visits I enjoyed shopping trips. Once, I accompanied my sister to return a couple of toasters. She received multiple models as engagement party gifts. She didn't need three of them so two had to go. With the store exchange she could fill in some items that remained on her wish list.

That excursion was different since it required stopping at destination stores in multiple strip malls. Large indoor malls require one in and out of a car trip. But strip mall destination stores mean in and out and in and out and in and out, again and again.

Poor Mair—she might have been able to complete her task in half the time if she had gone by herself. My special needs made every store we stopped at an event—if not a more like a duPont PT session.

She was a good sport about all the extra effort it took to literally drag me along on her errands. I honored her for loving me enough to take me—and not out of pity. With a thankful heart I welcomed the challenge knowing it could only strengthen my patience and personal discipline.

On one weekend home, Alan, Kris, Russ, and I planned a trip to the county fair, even though I couldn't go on any rides. I loved the fair and the rides were my favorite part.

That July, the fairgrounds looked much like it did every July when the annual event brought together people from all over South Jersey in celebration of farm and family. Youngsters displayed their handcrafted creations from sewing clubs to home economics to plant and farm husbandry in the 4-H exhibits featured in the great hall. The exhibits displayed club members' project work set against a backdrop tableau of clever themes. Illustrative posters, catchy slogans, and complex dioramas caught the eye like window dressings in great city department stores. They told stories or taught an element of something learned.

Being wheelchair bound at the fair for the first time, I found the exhibit hall more interesting than I ever had before. In the past, I made a beeline for the Midway where all the ride and arcade action was with barely a cursory walk through the exhibits.

But without the ability to take in Midway activities, I leisurely rolled through the hall and enjoyed what I'd always thought to be the most boring part of the fair.

But poor David. He squirmed and just wanted to be outside where he could run and see all the animals lined up in the rows of pens and stables.

The wheelchair was not a problem in the buildings with the displays, but the uneven ground carpeted in mounds of hay and dust did not accommodate the thin wheels of the chair I was strapped to. I slowed everyone down.

"I'm sorry. Stuck again."

Alan ran ahead with David while Kris and Russ helped me hobble over the ground on the smoothest surfaces they could find.

David loved the pigs best. I knew that's where they'd be when we got to the stables. And, of course, they happened to be in the muddiest part of the pens, so I kept getting stuck. "I'm sorry. Can you help me, Kris?"

"Don't keep apologizing, Paula." She took a firm hold of the chair and yanked to wrangle my wheels out of a muddy rut. "It is what it is."

"Why don't you just get me over to that dry area there. I'll wait til David gets his fill." I resolved not to rain on their parade and removed myself from the constant stopping and starting because of a clunky wheelchair. "I'll just watch from a distance."

"Are you sure?" Kris looked concerned.

"Yes. I'm good. Really. Just get me over there and you guys go see the animals with Alan and David. I'll be fine."

Kris did as I asked and gave me a funny, pouty look. "Here ya go. You sure you're okay?"

I bit my tongue, not wanting to blurt out something I'd regret at the sight of her pity-pout. I was determined to have a great day at the fair. "Kris—I'm fine. Now get!"

As I watched her leave with Russ to rendezvous with Alan, I could have shed a tear or two. But I was committed— no pity parties for me! I had to show people that I was tougher than that stupid old wheelchair. I'm glad I pushed back the urge to scold her for pouting at me. I didn't want her pity—but more so—I didn't want her pity to rub off on me or it might morph into my pity.

It's no matter. Next year I'll run in the mud with David and share pig snorts with him when the county fair comes to town again.

Growing up, anytime a Midway was nearby for a festival event, I was all in! Just put me on any ride and I was game for it. Especially the Zipper—a cage you strapped into that hydraulically lifted you high into the air. At full height, the cage dropped in a free spin, and you swirled in dizzy chaos to the bottom.

I tried to keep David still on my lap and waved at Alan, Kris, and Russ as they loaded onto the Zipper ride. I could only watch—hungry to be there and a part of all the fun. *Next year. Next. year.*

David got restless. "Look! Look, David! See Daddy all the way up there? Mommy is going to be up there next year! You'll see! You'll be so proud of your mommy!'

I wiped at moist eyes. *Just a bit of sand in my eye from when those teens ran close by and kicked up the dirt.*

Soon, we wandered into the arcade section of the grounds where I participated in some of the games. I showed off my arm strength and knocked down milk cans with expert ease. But the ring toss eluded my prowess because it was awkward to gently toss and target the bowling pins from my sitting position.

Eventually, I did ring one of the pins to enthusiastic applause. Maybe too enthusiastic. *Hey—don't treat me like I'm just too special with all your exaggerated congratulations for reaching the lowest goal.*

Even so, the people working the game awarded me with the big prize as if I'd made a ringer with every toss. I wanted to turn it away, but David quickly scooped up the giant stuffed Scooby Doo before I could open my mouth.

Okay. I'll take the win for David.

The next weekend, Dr. Haag came to the house to visit me—our family doctor and the first professional I saw when my nightmare began. He diagnosed me with a sinus infection at the time. "Incredible story, Paula. Incredible progress you're making."

We engaged in polite conversation for an hour, and he left. As mom shut the door behind him, she turned to me with a look of disdain. "You know, Paula, that guy was completely wrong about you when you first went to see him. He missed it entirely. What if he hadn't and got you to the hospital for tests right away instead of waiting until you were going into the coma?"

"I don't know, Mom. I don't think we can say it would have been much different. I did have a sinus infection. How could he have known the infection would travel the way it did?"

"Well, let me tell you what Gloria Palermo said about you maybe having a really good lawsuit on your hands with Dr. Haag."

"A lawsuit? Are you kidding?"

She sat down next to me wearing her serious look and took my head between her hands. "Paula, your insurance is paying for a lot, but we still don't know what our out-of-pocket bill will be when this is all said and done. You have to be honest about the kind of debt you may have in the long run."

Debt. I hadn't really thought about how much things cost. The money being spent to help me walk again and fully recover had not even entered my radar. Was I irresponsible to not think about how much money this whole ordeal would cost in the end?

Mom stroked my hair and lowered her voice. "Sweetheart, I know it's a lot to think about, but Gloria is not the only person to suggest suing Dr. Haag. I mean, we all like him, but you must admit, there could be a case here. He should have caught this."

I didn't agree. There was no one to blame. Except for the mosquito, of course. And it was long dead. I don't think they last more than a day after they've syphoned you.

I liked Dr. Haag. How could he have known what was going to happen to me? I just wanted to focus on getting my life back — my standing up, walking around, and moving on with my life-plan back.

A lawsuit against a well-liked doctor in our small town was a terrible idea. Mom and her friends were concerned about how I might pay for the additional hospital and therapy costs. But I couldn't think about such things at that time. *It's just another detail You'll have to handle for me, Lord. You've brought me this far. I can trust You for the rest of the journey.*

"No, Mom. I'll be fine. Poor Doc Haag — leave him be. C'est la vie."

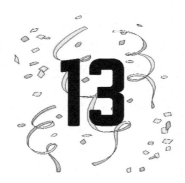

Back at duPont, my therapists said I mastered wheelchair trials with flying colors. I neglected to tell them about my splat in the parking lot.

Nurse and nurse assistant, Amy and Karen, arrived my first morning back after the mall visit weekend to shower me. I could only sponge bathe when I was home. They brought the special plastic wheelchair that looked like it was made of PVC pipes—specially designed for invalid showers.

After so many new milestones met and growing independence in many areas, my heart sank at the thought of showering as a threesome again. The humiliation of stripping down and having four foreign hands lather me up was something I'd never gotten used to.

Amy clearly saw the disappointment on my face and gently inquired, "Ready for your shower?"

"Yes. I suppose so. Let's get this over with." I positioned myself on my bed and plopped into the mesh seat of the shower chair while Karen held it in place.

It was an odd-looking chair with four small rubber tires about 8 inches in diameter and 3 inches thick; a no frills, simple framework chair designed to get wet and not rust.

Nurse and aide exchanged odd glances as we moved towards the door. I grabbed my toiletry bag and change of clothes on the way out and we wheeled down the hall to the shower room shared by all the patients on the floor.

The large room had four private square stalls, each about 8 feet wide which allowed plenty of room for a wheelchair and two shower aides. Amy grabbed the bath towel and washcloth from the table set just outside the stalls and wheeled me under the shower head. I placed my toiletry bag and fresh clothes on the wall hooks nearby.

Then to my surprise, Amy and Karen stepped away from the chair.

"Where are you going?"

"We'll be right outside here if you need us." Amy's grin could not be masked.

Is she teasing me?

"What do you mean? Aren't you giving me a shower?"

"Nope," Amy stepped to the other side of the marble stall threshold, "you're giving yourself a shower."

I paused a moment, trying to make sense of her words. "By myself?"

"All by yourself," Amy's eyes softened. She noticed my eyes begin to mist. "You can do it, Paula. You are such a champ." She nodded and looked at Karen. They left the room and closed the door shouting back, "Just yell if you need us."

I was speechless. I never thought I'd ever enjoy a just me shower again. But now I had to figure out how to do it in a clunky chair and half a working body. *How can I compensate?*

First—undress. From the waist up this was not a problem. However, wriggling out of my pants in a sitting position, with legs that didn't move with you as needed, presented a challenge. I leaned forward and scooched the pants around my bum, then rocked side to side inching them down bit by bit until I could toss them aside on the floor away from where the water would spray.

I reached over to where my toiletry bag hung, pulled out my soap and washcloth, sat back in all my glory and sighed. *Now what?*

Turn on the water, Paula!

Yes! Turn on the water. Isn't it funny how we take for granted the things we do without thinking day in and day out? I'd showered by myself since I was six years old. But, in that moment, I felt like a five-year-old wondering why mommy wasn't there to turn on the water and lather up the cloth, careful to make sure I didn't get soap in my eyes.

I lingered too long in preparation because I heard Amy call out, "You okay in there, Paula?"

"Yes! I'm fine. I just need to turn on the water, I guess." I heard snickering. *Is Amy pranking me?*

"Just turn the water on, Paula. You'll figure out the rest as you go along."

I rolled my eyes, leaned forward and set the water to warm, fearful I might scald myself if it was too hot. To my shock, it was not too hot. In fact, the first few seconds of water spurted out upon me like an arctic freeze. "Ahhhh!"

"You okay?"

"I'm good! I'm good! Just a polar bear plunge moment but the water's good now."

Snickering again. I'll bet Amy enjoyed my first foray into independent showering more than our midnight prank on Scott. I felt the distain he must have felt for being the subject of a bit of fun.

But, once the water settled to a tolerable temperature, it rolled over my shoulders and ran down my body. I melted into the comfort of it and lathered cucumber-melon body wash over my arms and down my legs. The finest spas on the French Riviera in all elegance and splendor could not have felt any better.

Back in my room, dressed in clean clothes, I stared out the window from my bed. *What an accomplishment today! My nurses will never share a shower stall with me again. Bravo, me!*

Independence Day! At least for showers.

No more humiliating arms flailing about me in all my nakedness. One less invalid checkmark on my chart. I wanted more.

As the days progressed, I surprised the aides with my bed made and room clean without them lifting a finger. "Whoa, Paula, this was on my work chart for today. Who did this?" Karen was out of a job.

I beamed a wide grin with boastful eyes. "I did it all by myself!"

Karen approved my efforts with a torrent of encouraging words. Nurse Paula arrived to see what the chatter was about. "You did your own room?"

"Yep!" I stood before them holding onto my walker and looked like I'd just discovered the cure for cancer or some other outrageous feat.

Then Paula looked at me with concern. "Why don't you have the sheet around your waist? You know that's the protocol for being up in your walker?"

I felt a little cocky. "Welp, I don't plan on falling down so you don't need that old sheet to grab onto to yank me off the floor."

Paula and Karen looked at each other then back to me. Karen moved to the closet to get a sheet and Paula gently scolded me for my oversight. And perhaps an ultra-cavalier attitude.

"Really. I'm good. I don't need that old sheet. I'm not going to fall. See?"

And then—I did it. I don't know why I did it. But I did. I thought I could—so I did.

I let go of the walker and stood. Alone. On my own two sneakered feet. I looked Paula in the eyes with all the confidence of an Olympic gold medal gymnast who just landed a triple flip off the balance beam with unparalleled precision.

We all stood, stunned at the sight of me standing with no support. For the longest two seconds in the world.

Then, my impression of Mary Lou Retton standing alone with her gold faded to just me, Paula. Aware that standing for three seconds might be pushing it a bit, I grabbed the walker and steadied myself. We sighed in relief—then broke into laughter and a few celebratory tears.

I stood.

If I can stand for two seconds today. I can stand for three tomorrow. And four the next day. And so on and so on. And then—I can walk!

That evening, I greeted my parent's visit sitting up in bed, just as they normally saw me. I tried to pretend that nothing unusual had happened that day, but it wasn't easy. Encouraged by my great feat from earlier in the day, I hatched a plan to surprise everyone. I didn't say anything about my accomplishment and had sworn the doctors and nurses to secrecy. "Don't tell my family! I want to surprise them."

For the next two days I worked my bum off to increase the amount of standing time without leaning on the walker. I perfected my steps with the walker to diminish dependency on my arm strength. Amazingly, my legs and feet responded to my will to walk.

Step by step, as I worked relentlessly, I grew confident to stand alone, strengthening my leg muscles so they didn't wobble like spaghetti noodles under me. I improved from morning to afternoon, to morning to afternoon. The staff eagerly followed my progress with amazement. Few patients that arrived at duPont with my type of diagnosis ever saw such positive gains with a hopeful prognosis.

Dr. Steg shook her head in wonder. "Paula, it's like you grow stronger by the hour!"

Did my will to walk impact my muscle memory and strength? Did Mom's eastern seaboard prayer effort turn the tide for healing? I had no clue. I just knew that by the end of the week when my parents visited, I couldn't hold back my excitement another minute.

"Mom! Dad! I have a surprise for you!" They arrived that evening to find me reading in bed.

"What is it? Did you make something in the craft class? You were getting good at the pottery making."

Mom would have continued discussing my experiments in clay if I hadn't cut her off. "No. Can you guys go in the hallway for a second?"

"The hallway—is it out there?"

"It will be. Just wait out where those chairs are near the nurse's station."

They obeyed and walked out of the room speculating about what the surprise could be and where they thought we were going.

Meanwhile, I rang for Nurse Amy. She was in on my plan, of course, and helped me with the protocol we'd agreed upon. She insisted I wear the sheet around my waist—just in case—and had made sure all the charts in sight of my family when they visited did not reveal the truth about my speedy progress that week.

I stood by my bed with the walker in place and started for the door. Amy swung the door wide open and my parents looked in to see me standing and walking without spaghetti noodle jerkiness. I walked slowly, but confidently. And as I came to the threshold of the door, I stood for a full four seconds, with my arms raised above my head in the shape of a V for Victory!

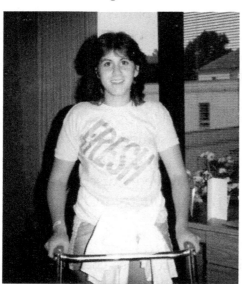

Tears streamed down my face in a rush of emotion. *Hold on to your hats, everybody . . . Look at me! I can move my legs! I can walk with a walker! Very slowly and clumsy, but I can walk! Only for a few short steps, but I can walk! Thank you, Jesus!*

Did you get that?
I could walk!

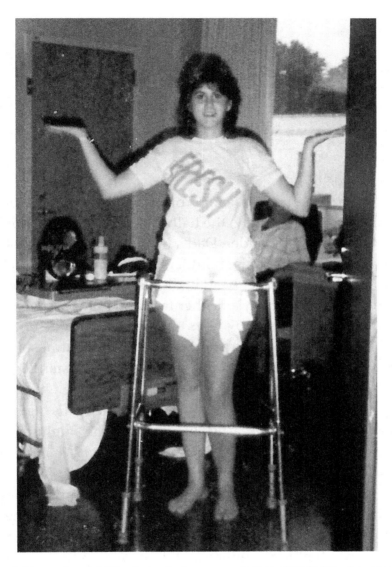

Look Ma, no hands! After I shocked my parents that night in late July showing them my new walking skills, we laughed more and talked about a bright future. No Hands was the goal for the rest of my life. Eventually I went from the walker to Canadian crutches, the kind that cuffs around your upper arm, to a simple cane. And then—just me and my legs the way God intended.

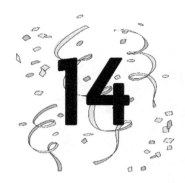

Time stood still.

Everyone in the vicinity of my room froze in place. Then, in perfect harmony, the hallway exploded into shouts of joy and gasps of wonder. Dad's wide eyes closed tight. He dropped his head and his shoulders heaved in thankful sobs of relief. Mom shook her head in disbelief for a fleet moment before she rushed to my side, her face and voice a jumble of joyful emotion and sloppy tears and praises to God.

Alan arrived later that evening to a party atmosphere in my room, shocked at what he saw. There I was standing— STANDING! "Surprise!"

He scooped me into his arms with one of his big bear hugs, then pulled back a bit, worried that he might break me. *No, babe. I won't break. I conquer mountains, remember?* There would be no pity party that night!

I did conquer mountains. Way back in summer camp, scaling those rocky trails year after year, and guiding others to do the same. That night I felt the same summer camp mountain climbing euphoria I'd known years before because I could stand and walk for a few seconds without crumpling to the ground.

After everyone left and the night lights came on, I lay wide-eyed in my bed thinking through the events of the day. *I did it! I did it!*

Something flickered above my head. A glimmer of light from the hallway reflected off the gold on the Rosary beads that had hung there for weeks. Mom placed them there along with a Catholic Scapula for Divine protection and as a reminder of the many friends and family praying for my recovery. Why should anyone then be surprised when I actually did recover?

I reached up and fingered the smooth cross over my head as the beads clicked against each other. I hadn't done anything on my own. Oh yes, I worked hard. Harder than anything I'd ever done. And the support of family and friends and hospital staff was irreplaceable.

But, if the Lord hadn't been with me like in the past when I walked on the mountain trails sensing His Presence, I knew I wouldn't be celebrating. God coached me like a loving and compassionate hiking partner, constant and true. He wanted me to succeed—just like I wanted Donna to succeed.

In my mind's eye I saw her again, staggering her way, huffing and puffing, up that old mountain trail as I coaxed her along in my last summer at camp. I refused to leave her behind. I refused to let her throw away all her future potential by failing in her trial.

In the same way, I realized that it wasn't just my hard-headed determination that brought me to my triumphant moment. God heard me cry out to Him for help on Independence Day and many frightful nights in my hospital bed when things seemed impossible to overcome. He met me in my need. He'd been there all the time, every minute. He never left—just like I never left Donna. Conquering mountains, the only thing we left behind was defeat.

"Good teamwork, God," I whispered, "between my hard head and You being . . . well . . . You . . . we did it!"

I wiped a tear, and a level of gratefulness flooded my heart as I'd never known before. God was real to me in the light of sunny skies on long ago mountain tops, and just as real in the dark of my hospital room that night.

Some years later, a friend told me about a Scripture in Psalm 139:1-11 NKJV that sums up what I lived through:

O Lord, You have searched me and known me.
You know my sitting down and my rising up;
You understand my thought afar off.
You comprehend my path and my lying down,
And are acquainted with all my ways.
For there is not a word on my tongue,
But behold, O Lord, You know it altogether.
You have hedged me behind and before,
And laid Your hand upon me.
Such knowledge is too wonderful for me;
It is high, I cannot attain it.
Where can I go from Your Spirit?
Or where can I flee from Your presence?
If I ascend into heaven, You are there;
If I make my bed in hell, behold, You are there.
If I take the wings of the morning,
And dwell in the uttermost parts of the sea,
Even there Your hand shall lead me,
And Your right hand shall hold me.
If I say, "Surely the darkness shall fall on me,"
Even the night shall be light about me;

I didn't really think of it that way then. I only knew God had been with me, just like the Scriptures promised, all the time.

I fingered the smooth lacquer of the crucifix again. The gentle click-clacking of the beads sounded like melodious wind-chimes tinkling in a soft summer breeze. In that instant, life and hope filled me to overflowing. Tomorrow would be the beginning of the end as the doctors announced my discharge date: August 8—less than 4 weeks away!

Immediately, PT sessions increased in intensity. I worked my legs harder and didn't need assistance to move them. It felt more like working out in a gym with a personal trainer, not a physical therapist. I grew in strength and more life skill exercises were added to my muscle building routine.

Ascending and descending stairs presented a challenge. There were only three of them with railings on both sides. At first, I was dependent on those railings and could only manage it with a step-step—both feet, one step at a time. But before I knew it, I advanced to step-step-step-step—one step and one foot at a time.

All that working out required a fair amount of food to keep me going. My appetite was on steroids. I ate anything and everything set before me. Bring on the meatballs and pasta from home, and I welcomed cakes, snacks, pizza, burgers—you name it, I ate it. Fuel for all the calories I burned every day. My sleep was sound and as I checked off the days on the calendar through July, my anticipation for release day grew.

The doctors greeted me daily with exclamations of wonder. Not one of them thought I would ever recover the use of my legs, let alone advance in recovery at warp speed. I continued to enjoy regular visits with family and friends and the active planning of what to do once I got home.

I was a bridesmaid in three weddings within the next few months—the first of which would be in September for my friend Debbie Harris. I loved chatting with her about all the wedding plans and was thankful that I would be home in time for her bridal shower. I never wanted to miss a good party!

I also made sure to spend time with the friends I'd made at duPont. Sometimes, I was able to help them with a little chore here or there because I'd regained movement and ability. Everyone was glad for me as I grew stronger, and I marveled at the selfless way they cheered me on in my efforts.

Scott, of the Midnight Nail Polish Caper fame, sometimes appeared to be happy for me. But on occasion, I caught a telling expression on his face as he watched me walk into the cafeteria. Words didn't need to be exchanged. I felt his pain. My bedridden friend had his own mountains to climb, but did he have a coach to guide him through treacherous terrain? His injuries were more extreme than mine. I wonder, after all these years, how his journey worked out.

Busy days, every day, revolved around not just my PT regimen, social visits, and eating, but with preparations for my departure. I started a list of things to do before I left, not the least of which was to choose a fashionable outfit to wear on the big day.

I dreamt about wearing something dressy, but in reality, we were working class folk, so I resorted to cute baggy cotton pants, and a button down top. I did, however, have a new pair of sneakers, and the hairdresser in me made sure my brown locks looked fabulous and my makeup applied with cover girl perfection.

The morning of August 8th arrived with sunlight streaming through the window. Of course, it would be sunshine and blue skies! No pity parties or rain on my parade that day.

There seemed a lot of traffic in my room that morning. All the doctors stopped by for a final word and paperwork to be signed. The nurses and therapists on duty made sure to peek in with well wishes and a hug.

Saying goodbye to bestie Nurse Amy was hard. "What am I going to do without my midnight partner in pranks?" she whined at me as we squeezed hands and blinked back tears.

"Amy—you've got this! Find the craziest nail polish color and choose your victims well! You can do this!" We broke into laughter and another hug.

"I'm so proud of you, Paula," she whispered in my ear. "I will miss you so much."

I promised I'd be back to visit, and she threatened me with a drive all the way to New Jersey to prank me if I didn't.

Mom and Dad arrived with Alan, and we couldn't keep a straight face if we tried. Huge smiles seemed permanently plastered from cheek to cheek, and the adrenaline flowed through us all, electrifying the room with excitement.

"I'm going home!" I'd have jumped up and down like when I bowled a strike if I could have done so with elegance. I had more strength to build before I could leap like a confident gazelle again.

Alan and Dad grabbed my suitcases and left the room. Mom hugged me and looked me in the eye with a mix of pride and relief. I didn't appreciate then what it must have been like for her to see her baby girl lying in bed all those weeks, hearing dire predictions from doctors and experts about a stunted hope and future for me. *But, oh—how I can appreciate the emotional roller coaster she must have endured that summer of 1986, now!*

"You know, Paula," she said as we stood alone in my empty room but for the bed and machines I didn't need anymore, "I remember telling the doctors, 'There's no way Paula is going to spend her life in a wheelchair.' I said you would surprise them all—you'd never give in. I admit, I wasn't convinced during the first four weeks that you'd actually walk, but after that day you called us with your surprise, I knew you'd be your old self in no time."

"Well, I had to be able to walk in Debbie's wedding next month." I tried not to sound as emotional as I felt.

"Of course! And dance!" Her eyes caught something behind me. She stepped to the bed and reached over to the wall. "The Rosaries and Scapula!"

"Oops! Almost forgot those!"

Mom gently removed them from their perch where she had placed them weeks ago over my head. "Oh, we can't forget them. We can't forget all the people praying that they represent." She pursed her lips and dropped her head, choking back tears again. "Paula, when you first went to Elmer, they told us that we could lose you. But God had a miracle planned for you."

We hugged again and I fought back the tears. I'd labored over my makeup and didn't want it messed before I made my long-awaited exit. "We'd better go."

Mom tried to pick up my personal items, but I stopped her. "Nope! I'll carry them." I slung my backpack purse over my right shoulder and picked up the large paper sack brimming with "get well" cards and gifts with that hand, then grabbed my Vineland Academy of Beauty makeup and hair box with my left hand. "Let's go!"

Leaving my room for the last time was bittersweet. It had been my home for quite a while. As we walked out the door, I looked back at the bare bone furnishings. The important moments I'd experienced there flashed through my mind in an instant like a movie preview. I held the memory tight, then tucked it safely away and turned to face the hall.

As I walked out, doctors, nurses, therapists, and patients lined the corridor. I'd grown to love and regard many of them as friends. Everyone clapped for me, as if I were some sort of a celebrity—an awkward feeling since I wasn't one who loved the spotlight.

Even so, I was proud of myself and accepted the cheers and applause but wished the other patients could walk alongside me. One step at a time, I laughed, nodded, waved, and thanked everyone along the way.

I saw Scott. He was elevated in his bed, tucked close to a wall as I passed by. Like Dorothy would miss Scarecrow the most, I would miss Scott the most. He and I became more than friends. We were each other's shoulder to cry on. Who would he depend on to make his toes look pretty and whoop him in Scrabble? He smiled as I walked by him and would have waved if he could raise his arm.

Soon we were at the front door of the hospital where I'd arrived two months earlier by ambulance. As I drew close to the large glass doors with no walking aid, I felt kind of naked—like I'd forgotten something. But I continued, triggered the sensor, and the doors swung open wide. I felt the breeze of a beautiful summer day sweep across my face and crossed the threshold of duPont to freedom. Dad waited outside with his Kodak 110 camera to capture the moment forever.

On Independence Day, after God and I came to an understanding—ahem—I resolved to walk out of the hospital on my own power. And I did.

Happy chatter celebrating my miracle recovery peppered the forty-minute drive home. But my mind buzzed with expectation of some unfinished business ahead.

David. David. I have to get David! Those were the last words I spoke as I lay helpless on the floor of my bedroom after my legs collapsed and my nightmare began.

I promised to get David from his room to start the day, and once the car pulled into our driveway that's precisely what I did when I crossed the threshold of my own home two months later. I walked into David's room, bent down from a standing position, and hugged my baby boy.

"Mommy's home!" he shouted—and squeezed my neck with an embrace I will never forget.

"Yes, baby!" I squeezed him back. "Mommy's home."

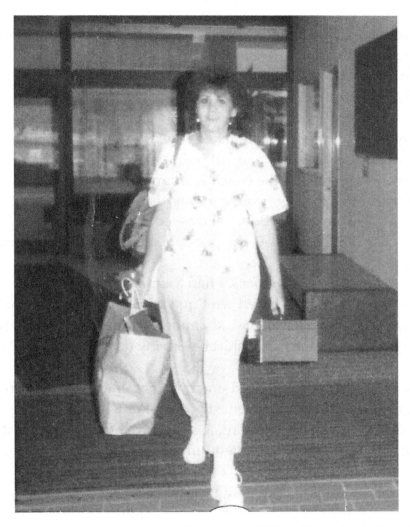

I told you I would walk out of here! On August 8, 1986, I did exactly what I said I would do—I walked out of that hospital on my own two feet by my own power. Praise the Lord! They said it couldn't be done, but I showed 'em good! I felt great and with all the workout I'd been doing, was a tall, svelte size 10 looking forward to some disco dancing soon.

Epilogue

I looked at my Swatch watch and readjusted David on my lap as he fingered the smooth clock face on my wrist. *Russ and Kris will be here soon. How much longer is this guy gonna stay? Haven't we answered enough questions?*

Bob Shryock of the *Gloucester County Times* sat in the green chair near the kitchen doorway with his pencil scribbling words on a small spiral bound notebook. I sat across from him on the couch as mom paced from kitchen to living room playing hostess to our visitor.

"More coffee, Bob?" she asked.

"No. Thank you. I'm good. Just a few more questions here."

A few more questions. I had a squirmy two-year-old on my lap who was as bored with questions as I was. The clock had just chimed half past six and I still needed to fix my makeup and change my shirt before my date at 7:00 p.m. *No more questions!*

But Mother chatted on about her emotional ups and downs regarding my recent stay at duPont. I played a finger weaving game to entertain David and hoped he'd settle down for the night. I wanted him to be ready for bed before I had to leave.

"Sounds like quite a miracle recovery. Great story!" The reporter jotted a few more notes and requested clarification on a couple of points. I watched the clock tick. He'd been there for over an hour and though I was honored to be interviewed for a feature story in the *Gloucester County Times*, I needed to move on with my evening plans. The Franklinville Roller Rink awaited my grand entrance—the first such excursion there since my return from duPont.

146

Mom gave a great interview. She welcomed this local celebrity status with the miraculously healed daughter the experts said would never walk again. Over the past few weeks, our home received a constant stream of friends, family, and well-wishers bringing meals and gifts, eager to see me walk across the room. Or scale the stairs. Or swim in the pool. Whole and hearty again.

I enjoyed the attention for a bit but was ready to move on and put my ordeal behind me. There were weddings forthcoming, my graduation from beauty school, and an active life to fully embrace.

There were also many follow-up visits to the doctors for a few issues that remained to be dealt with as an out-patient.

My left ankle never quite healed completely. I walked on the outside of my foot. This required extra therapy for several years and recently, some 40 years after the fact, my ankle was surgically rebuilt. Seventy-one staples secured four distinct cuts by the able hand of Dr. Brian Winters of the Rothman Institute in Egg Harbor Township, New Jersey. Therapy continued after that, too, with a perfect outcome.

As I've aged, my body has changed in many ways and minor issues that remained after duPont grew into greater issues that needed to be addressed anew.

The nerves to my bladder never healed 100 percent. Doctors tried everything they could think of to remedy this embarrassing issue until my family doctor, Dr. Brian Davis, recommended me to a specialist with a unique cure.

He introduced me to the idea of a mechanical insert for the bladder—sort of like a pacemaker for the heart. In this case, it pulses a signal from my bladder to my brain to make me aware that I have to go to the bathroom. In effect, an artificial nerve. I've lived with this little friend I call my "pee machine" since mid-life—for the past twelve years, as of this writing.

Before this miracle procedure, I endured a constant state of incontinence and couldn't go anywhere beyond my house without an embarrassing episode. Many thanks to Dr. Gary Mirone of the Jane Osborne Center for Women's Health in Cape May Courthouse, New Jersey, for giving me another new lease on life.

Thankfully, my healing after duPont was complete until these later in life concerns—not unlike any one of us developing arthritis or joint strain from an active lifestyle. I approached these minor setbacks with the same resolve my nineteen-year-old self attacked that dire diagnosis in 1986.

Back to my living room interview with Mr. Shryock, I worked out how quickly I'd have to dress and rush my makeup and became aware of heightened voice volume.

"Paula, Mr. Shryock asked you a question." Mom stepped to my side and lifted David from my lap.

"Oh! I'm sorry. Can you repeat that?"

The reporter turned to face me more direct and smiled. Did he know he had overstayed his time? "Do you feel you can participate in some of the same activities you used to, or are there some things you can't do anymore."

What a great question! Now I have a door of escape! I wasted no time in my response. "Well, one of my favorite activities is roller skating and . . . oh! Look at the time! I just happen to be heading out in a few minutes to the roller rink with my friends. I need to excuse myself and get David settled so I'm not late."

I stood and took David back into my arms.

Mr. Shryock stood and apologized for keeping us so long.

Mom apologized for having to cut the interview short due to my—ahem—active social life. Poor Mom. She'd never been interviewed for the newspaper before and was soaking in every moment of the honor.

When the article appeared in the newspaper with a terrific picture of me and David, plus copious quotes from Mom, it was clear he had gathered plenty of information.

My celebrity status got another boost and another round of well wishes followed. Not the least of which was from our Assemblyman at the time, Jack Collins. An anonymous fan forwarded the newspaper article to him. He sent me a personal letter and State of New Jersey citation of honor for my birthday a couple of months later.

I often wondered about the way people reacted to my recovery—how joyfully they interacted with me in a celebratory spirit. Even complete strangers, upon hearing my story of despair rising to victory on the wings of prayer and resilience absorbed the details of my ordeal with rapt attention. As though they were trying to sift through my experience to inform something needy in their experience.

How could I have inspired others had I capitulated to the initial diagnosis and resigned myself to that bed in duPont? In defeat, I could not have been the example God wanted me to be of His goodness and love towards us all.

"We rejoice in our sufferings, knowing that suffering produces endurance, and endurance pro-duces character, and character produces hope, and hope does not put us to shame, because God's love has been poured into our hearts . . . "

Romans 5:3-5 ESV

I've heard it said that God doesn't give us more than we can handle. He gives us all we can handle in the sufficiency of His Grace and faithfulness to complete the work He has begun in us.

Thinking back to my days of trail walking in the mountains I best heard God's voice when I'd sit alone in His Presence in Creation. I know He planted something strong and courageous within my spirit in those days. But if it was really all about me being strong and courageous, would I have overcome to enjoy a restored life? In hindsight, the gift of resilience, strength, and courage found their full portion when I pushed them to the limit. God made up the rest and multiplied my efforts.

My life looked hopeless for a season—as good as dead to a young, energetic kid with her whole life ahead of her. I could have given up—but my Heavenly Coach refused to leave me to crash on that mountain when He called me forward to the top. When I was weak, He was strong. One step at a time, I learned the goodness of God is enough to scale any mountain.

And that's where the real shindig is! No pity party for me. I live to celebrate life and the goodness of God every day.

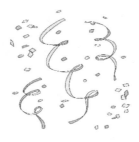

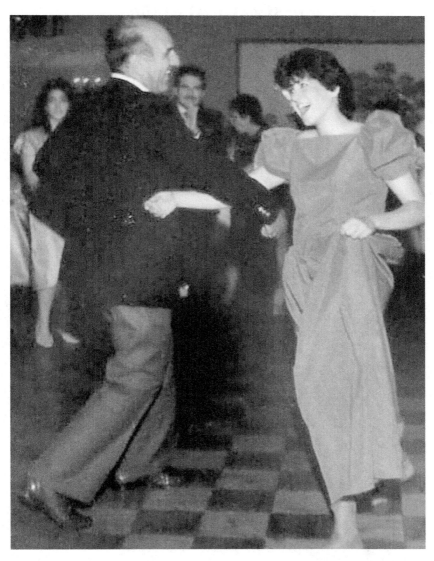

And so, I DANCED at Marianne and Dean's wedding with cousin Alfred! Just a few months before, at their engagement party, my troubles began with that mosquito bite. The dire prognosis was not to be. I couldn't have been happier than stomping on that dance floor like I was stomping on the devil who tried to keep me strapped in a wheelchair. You betcha! No pity parties for me!

PHOTO ALBUM

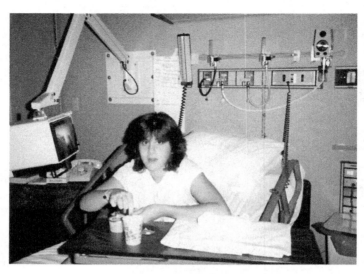

Sorting my vitamins to get ready for another week of hard work in PT. I looked forward to some TV on the large crane arm to my right. The sheets on the table were to tie around my waist when I used the walker. In case I fell it was easier for the nurses to grab hold to hoist me up.

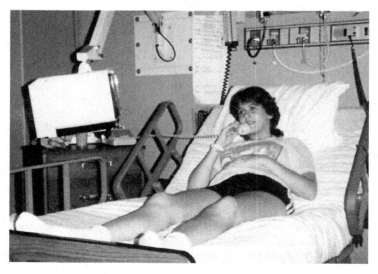

Every morning, I looked forward to my call with David, then watched the Today Show on the TV to catch up on what was going on in the world. I was always so happy and thankful to hear my bright-eyed boy's voice in the morning!

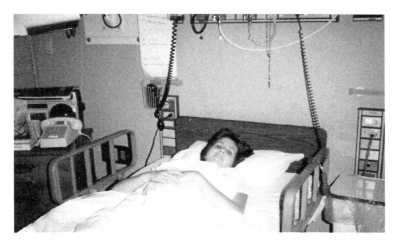

I'm ready for a good night sleep on June 23, 1986. The TV is stowed above, and Dean lent me the boom box on the bed table. He made me cassette music of all the top 40 hits like Madonna and Michael Jackson. The paper on the wall behind me was a schedule of new activities after some early signs of movement.

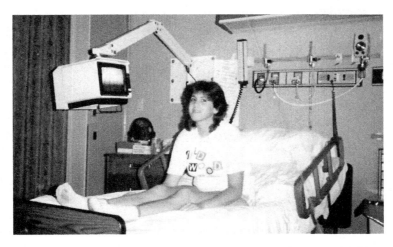

Okay. Let's get this day started—which included catheterizing myself. The round dark thing on my nightstand is the mirror I used to stand up in the bed so I could see what I was doing.

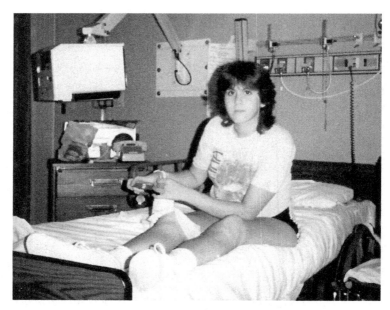

I pushed my own chair and got filthy hands from touching the wheels. Wet wipes were the first order of business after wheelchair time.

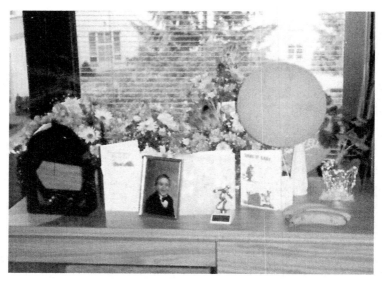

My room décor on the dresser in front of the big window featured David's portrait, my bowling trophy, cards from well-wishers and flowers.

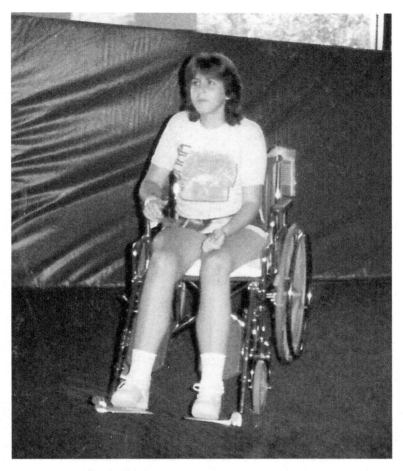

Left alone for a moment, someone caught me on camera in the rec room, looking on from a distance at my family and visitors having a good time. I loved playtime with David in the rec room when he came. I can see a bit of envy in my eyes that the chair restricted me from standing around, picking David up, or playing on the floor with him like everyone else could. At that point in my recovery, I had experienced some minor movement but had a long road ahead of me before I could enjoy freedom again. What I didn't know at the time, is how soon that early July day would be to the day I walked out of duPont on my own power.

THE ASSEMBLY
STATE OF NEW JERSEY
TRENTON

ASSISTANT MAJORITY WHIP
JACK COLLINS
ASSEMBLYMAN 3RD DISTRICT
SALEM-CUMBERLAND-GLOUCESTER COUNTIES
65 EAST AVENUE
WOODSTOWN, NJ 08098
609-769-9093
609-769-9093

COMMITTEES
VICE-CHAIRMAN
ECONOMIC DEVELOPMENT
& AGRICULTURE
MEMBER, HIGHER EDUCATION &
REGULATED PROFESSIONS

December 2, 1986

Ms. Paula Leone Aron
R.D. #4, Box 179
Elmer, New Jersey 08318

Dear Paula,

As you come down from your happiest Thanksgiving
and prepare for your happiest birthday, please allow me to
offer my best wishes.

The story of your successful effort to walk again,
which highlighted your positive determination was a
definite pick-me-up for me and my family.

I thank you for allowing all of us to share in your
"miracle." I'm sure that you, Allan and David are as
excited about life as any family in America.

I wish all of the Aron's the happiest of holiday
season's, and if I can ever be of assistance, please do
not hesitate to call me.

Sincerely,

Jack Collins
Assemblyman
3rd District

JC:vh
Enclosure

In November of 1986, Bob Shryock of the Gloucester County Times interviewed me and my family about our experience. He called it a miracle and wrapped his story around my recovery from something all the doctors said I'd never recover from. After the newspaper published the article, I received this beautiful letter commending me on my victory from then Assemblyman Jack Collins. When I found it in the mailbox, I had no idea why I'd be getting an official letter from a political leader. I received it the week of my birthday and thought it was great timing--another special moment to be thankful for that came out of something I thought I could never be thankful for. God has a way of turning darkness into light. My miracle recovery and the love I felt from family, friends, strangers, and even government leaders were a divine light that touched my heart in ways I still can't fathom.

About the Authors

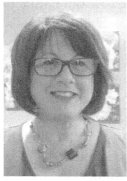

Paula Leone Heuling's amazing story of resilience and miraculous healing in a test of her faith and will to live a vibrant life has inspired her friends and family for decades. In the face of negative authoritative predictions, Paula and her family felt the embrace of their community and the effectiveness of prayer to buoy hope with steadfast courage.

After her discharge from duPont, Paula returned as a volunteer and worked with many of the patients she used to know on a resident peer level.

As the years passed, Paula's life journey blossomed in her career and family, even as it had setbacks and discouraging changes in fortune. Like all our lives, seasons of plenty and pain pepper our days on the earth. She met each as another mountain to scale or celebratory party to revel in.

She graduated from the Vineland Academy of Beauty in January of 1988 and has enjoyed a robust career in the beauty industry for over 3 decades, currently working for Contemporary Hair Designs in Vineland, New Jersey.

David welcomed a new baby brother, Gregory, in 1996. Both boys are grown and pursuing successful careers in culinary science and computers, respectively. Paula delights in her "Mammy" duties to David's three small children, Sophia, Landry, and Emmitt and shares in active sports with them like swimming and bike riding.

She married Otley in 2004, building a home together with their four-footed baby, Bailey, a 50-pound Irish Setter with delusions of being a Yorkshire Terrier lapdog. When the grandkids come to play with "Popot," he's ready for anything Paula and the kids dream up. Usually, it's some sort of adventure where they practice Paula's legacy of facing all things with courage and resolve.

As the years passed, a new dream stirred within Paula: to write and publish a book about her experience. She dreamed of telling her story to a broader audience and hoped to encourage others to persevere in dark times and contend for a life of celebration in victory—not pity parties in defeat.

In 2011, Paula finally put pencil to paper on the lined pages of a marble composition book and jotted down the details of her sickness and healing days at duPont. But her life, filled to the brim with child rearing and growing a successful business as a hairstylist, left her precious little time to make her dream as a writer come true. And, as the years passed, the cloudy details of those long-ago days receded into forgotten corridors of her memory. Would she ever have enough material to qualify as a book?

But in 2020, through an associate at the salon where she worked, Paula met author and independent publisher, Kathryn Ross. She handed the marble composition book with her scant recall of details, a handful of photographs, and a newspaper clipping to Kathryn and asked for a professional opinion on the feasibility of a book project.

The finished work you see here is the result.

A Note from Kathryn Ross

After months of digging into her past through my probing questions, Paula's mind reawakened long lost memories. She realized the full impact of varied life episodes she previously thought unrelated.

God's story in and through Paula's story surfaced alive with fresh illumination! The collaborative writing process tied together the chapters in her life with the cord of Christ's constancy, love, protection, and provision. Tears of joy and amazement were shared by both of us along the way.

From that young girl basking in His presence on the mountain trails, to the young wife and mother fighting to live her best life in the face of negative earthly odds, to the grandmother passing the torch of resilience and faith to this next generation — God has been ever present in Paula's life. His angels, though she may have been unaware, walked with her day by day. Night by night.

God was and continues to be active in Paula's life, coaching her to scale every rocky peak that juts into her life path as if to block her forward mobility.

Like Paula's victory story, and her own experience coaching Donna up that mountain trail in her teenage years, God does the same for each of us, though we don't always recognize it. He leads us onward and upward to conquer the mountains in our life that threaten to cast us down in defeat.

Our Christian faith speaks greater things. We are wise to look up, where we find Hope that anchors our soul firm and secure. Anchored in Him through craggy terrain, we shall not fall. (Hebrews 6:19)

Then, no matter the trail or trial, all life paths end in a victory party. Hardship conquered. God glorified. Lives changed. Fortunes restored. Dreams fulfilled. And, in such a way of life, as Paula said in our first meeting, "There's just no room for pity parties!"

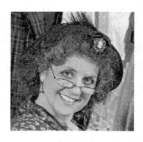 **Kathryn Ross** is a writer, speaker, dramatist, and teacher who equips women and families with the tools to develop a Family Literacy Lifestyle, producing readers and thinkers who can engage their world from a biblical perspective. She owns Pageant Wagon Publishing with book shepherd and publishing services for Christian writers and is the author of *The Gatekeeper's Key, Fragrant Fields: Poetic Reflections for Journaling,* and *Fable Springs Parables Picture Books,* among others. She lives in southern New Jersey with her book-seller husband Ed, in a house full of props, costumes, and bookshelves. To learn more about Miss Kathy and Pageant Wagon Publishing books and editing/publishing services, visit:

www.pageantwagonpublishing.com

Additional copies of this book are available in the Pageant Wagon BOOKSHOP:

www.pageantwagonpublishing.com/pageant-wagon-bookshop

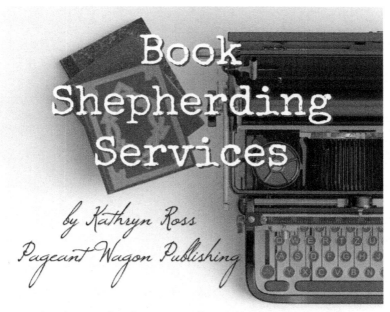

Book Shepherding Services

by Kathryn Ross
Pageant Wagon Publishing

Let me help you develop the book
God is calling you to write ~

From Idea to Finished Product!

A la carte and bundle services
include:
~ Monthly Consulting Sessions
~ Editing
~ Layout & Design
~ Print Publishing
~Audio Book Recording
~ Ghostwriting

www.pageantwagonpublishing.com

Made in the USA
Middletown, DE
18 August 2021

45328352R00096